JOAN'S WAY

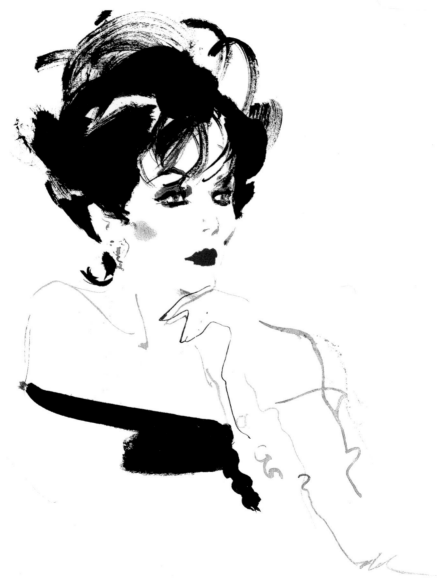

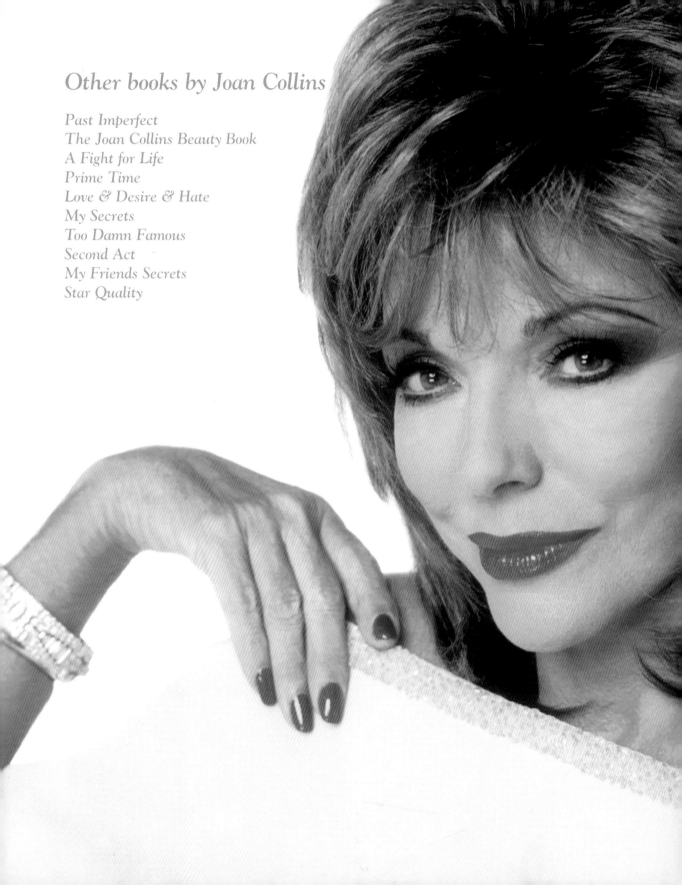

Other books by Joan Collins

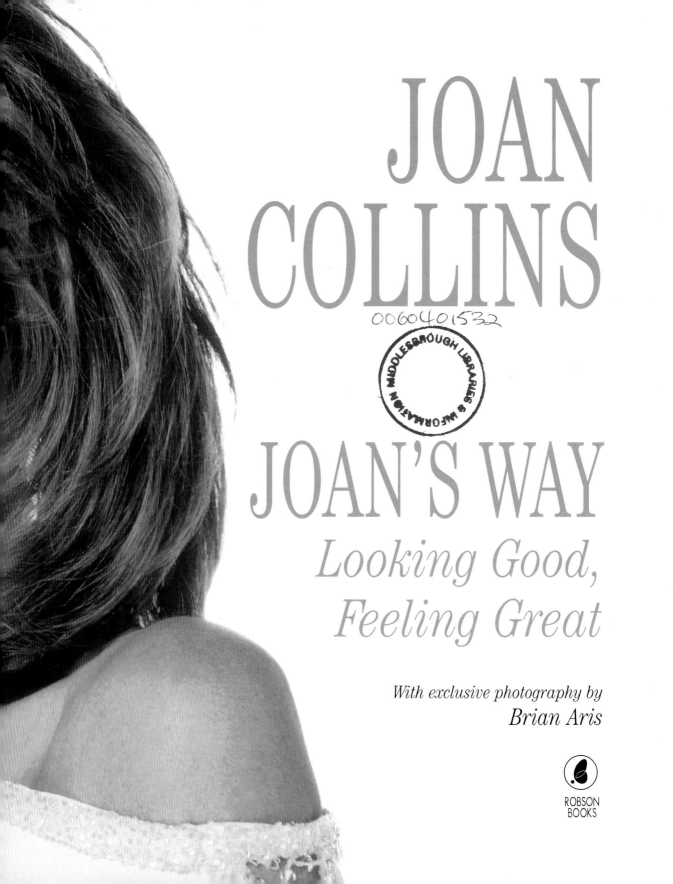

JOAN COLLINS

JOAN'S WAY

*Looking Good,
Feeling Great*

With exclusive photography by
Brian Aris

ROBSON
BOOKS

For Tara, Katy, Miel and Angela - The next dynasty

First published in Great Britain in 2002 by Robson Books, 64 Brewery Road, London,
N7 9NT

A member of Chrysalis Books plc

British Library Cataloguing in Publication Data
A catalogue record for this title is available from the British Library.

ISBN 1 86105 545 5

Designed by Ian Hughes, Mousemat Design
www.mousematdesign.com

Printed in Spain

While every effort has been made to ensure that the information is correct at the time
of going to press, the information in this book is for information only. It is not intended
as a substitute for the advice and guidance of a qualified health professional. If in doubt,
seek medical advice.

Neither the author nor the publisher can accept responsibility for any accident, injury
or damage that results from using the ideas, information or advice offered in this book.

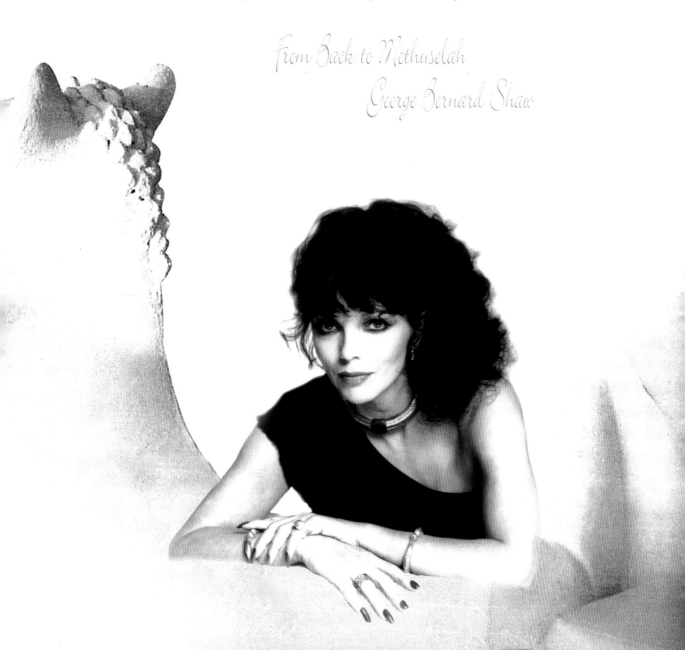

You see things and you say, 'Why?'
But I dream things and I say, 'Why not?'

From Back to Methuselah
George Bernard Shaw

Contents

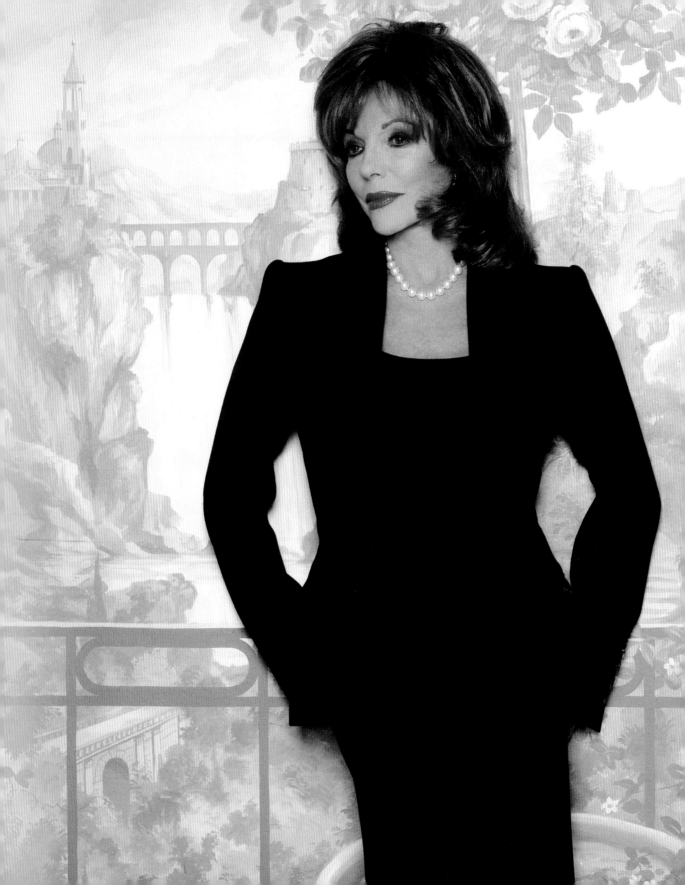

Prologue

Life isn't a rehearsal. How many times have we heard that old chestnut? It's become almost as much of a cliché as 'at the end of the day' and 'you know what I mean,' but the facts are true.

Life *isn't* a rehearsal, but it is *your* life and as it's the only one you're going to have, it's time to start taking care of your inner and outer self now. Exercising, eating properly and trying to rid yourself of those negative feelings that so many people allow themselves to indulge in is the start of a programme to make yourself feel and look better.

Sometimes I look back on the last 30 or 40 years of my life and I am astounded at how quickly it's sped by. And that's the problem. Unless we take the time and energy to enjoy each day fruitfully and, as much as we possibly can, happily, time just flies and often we have too little to show for it except for a few memories.

One of my close friends, the songwriter and lyricist Leslie Bricusse, has a wonderful philosophy about his life:

'I try to make each day a miniature lifetime in which I achieve something and I enjoy something.' Well, that may be tough for most people to achieve every day, although I know Leslie does, but I do believe that a healthy, productive and enjoyable life is a gift that sadly, we all too often don't appreciate or celebrate enough.

Celebrate yourself: don't just sit back and let your life drift by. Squeeze the most out of every day, whether it's by savouring your first cup of tea or coffee in the morning, buying a sinful packet of chocolate cookies, watching the early morning news (and comparing your life favourably to those less fortunate), hugging your loved one, taking a delicious scented bath, or looking out of the bus window at the fascinating passing parade of people.

Try to step back sometimes and appreciate the smaller things in life that can add up to a wonderful whole. When you wake up and stretch, feel how your whole body responds and enjoys the flexing and use of those muscles. Really stretch – copy a cat, they know how to do it. Smell the coffee. Yes, it's a great smell. Laugh at a cartoon in your daily paper or relish that first bite of toast and jam. There are so many little things that we enjoy but just take for granted.

There's a wonderful line in an old Humphrey Bogart movie, 'Live fast, die young and leave a good-looking corpse'. I'll go along with the first and the last phrase but no one wants to die young. The Bible tells us that three score years and ten is our allotted time span. Well, I'm greedy. I want a lot more lifetime than that, but it's got to be the *right* kind of life. Quality always wins over quantity and existing with pain and illness in the latter years is, I hope, not for me. Consequently, since my mid-twenties, I've realised that to be fully productive and happy, you have to be healthy on the outside *and* the inside, and much of that comes from how you go about the business of living through your attitude, optimism and daily routine.

No one gives you lessons in how to do this. My life lessons, as with most of my generation, were learned from my parents and I must admit that some of them were pretty good. Parents then were much more concerned about correct eating habits, daily exercise, good health and good manners than some of today's parents. Strangely enough, even with all the information available today, too many parents don't seem to have the child-rearing know-how that my mother and my grandmothers possessed. How did they know greens were good for you? Why did they insist on us being out in the open air, playing or doing gymnastics every day? Why did they stress that discipline, self-control and manners were an essential part of a well-rounded human being? But they did and their legacies have been invaluable to people like me, who see life as a series of obstacles that one must find the right tools to overcome.

In this book I'm going to share with you some of my life experiences and methods that will show you the way to feel better about yourself, and consequently you will look better. It isn't just about the physical though. I want to share with you some of the secrets of my lifestyle and reveal to you the choices that can be made. Entertaining friends, whether it's a wedding or tea for two, is one of life's most rewarding pleasures and I write about this in some detail. Love and relationships are also topics that make us tick as people and when these are fulfilling, they contribute tremendously towards achieving a more rounded and more productive life. A recent report revealed that women of 'un certain age' as the French say are happier than ever before. They're more independent, and experiencing richer relationships with husbands, lovers, family and friends.

Looking forward to a rosy future and a good third act!

While I can't pretend I'm an expert on all things – tattoos and belly button piercing are a mystery to me – I have learned much in my life, through my work and in my travels, and from this I believe I can benefit you, the reader. At least, I certainly hope so!

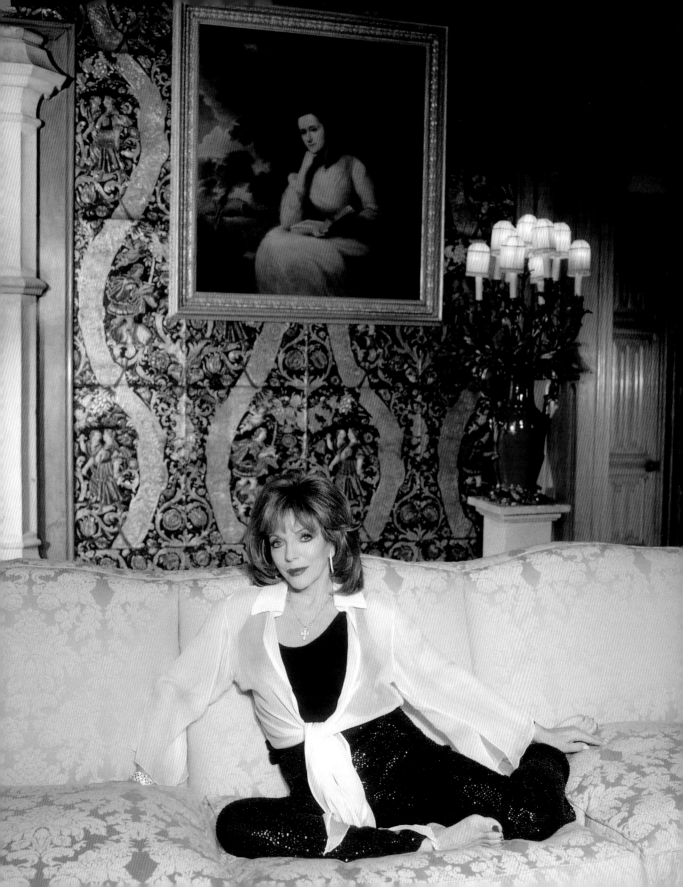

Introduction

My generation must have seen more change than any other in history. We were born before television, before penicillin, polio shots, frozen food, Xerox, plastic, contact lenses, videos, Frisbees or the Pill. We were born before radar, credit cards, split atoms, laser beams, CDs and ballpoint pens; before dishwashers, tumble dryers, electric blankets, air conditioners, drip-dry clothes and long before man first walked on the moon. We married first and *then* lived together. We thought fast food was what you ate during Lent, a Big Mac was an oversized raincoat and 'crumpet' was what you had for tea. We existed before househusbands, computer dating and dual careers in a time when a 'meaningful relationship' meant getting along with your cousins. 'Sheltered accommodation' was a place where you waited for a bus and 'politically incorrect' was when your local politician screwed up.

We were before day care centres, group homes and disposable nappies; we had never heard of FM radio, tape decks, electric typewriters, artificial hearts, word processors, computers, yoghurt or young men wearing earrings. For us 'time-sharing' meant togetherness, a 'chip' was a piece of wood or a fried potato; 'hardware' meant nuts and bolts, 'software' was pyjamas and a 'mouse' a scary little rodent. 'Made in Japan' often meant junk and the phrase 'making out' referred to how you did in your exams; 'stud' was something that fastened a collar to a shirt and 'going all the way' meant staying on the train to the end of the line. Pizzas, McDonalds, KFC and instant coffee were unheard of, cigarette smoking was fashionable, grass was mown, 'coke' kept in the coal house; a 'joint' was a piece of meat you had on Sundays and 'pot' was something you cooked in; 'rock music' meant a lullaby, a 'gay' person was the life and soul of the party, while 'aids' simply meant helping someone in trouble.

Debbie Reynolds, Elizabeth Taylor, Shirley Maclaine and I strut our stuff in the movie These Old Broads. *In spite of the ghastly title, we had a ball during filming.*

When you think of how the world has changed and the adjustments we've had to make, my generation must be a hardy bunch. Just look at Goldie Hawn, Cher, Sophia Loren, Judi Dench, Dolly Parton, Julie Christie, Helen Mirren, Diane Keaton, Tina Turner, Shirley Bassey, the list is endless. No wonder we are sometimes confused, but by the grace of God we *have* survived – and we're getting better and better.

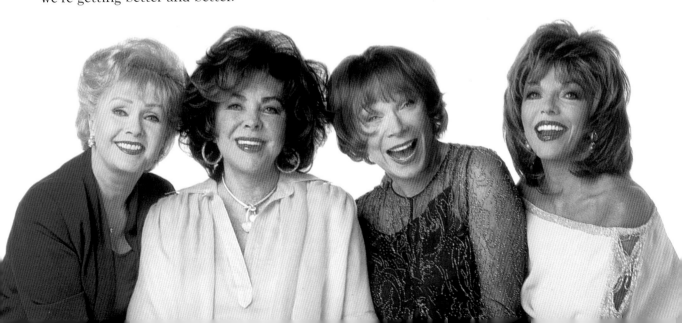

You're as young as you look

Think young, live young, forget the word 'old'

I never give my own age much thought. Whenever I see it printed in a newspaper, I subconsciously think, that can't be right, it's impossible. You see I truly believe you are as young as you look and feel. However much some journalists may criticise me, I know that I look, feel and behave several decades younger than my actual age and much of that is because I believe you are what you *think* you are. This is called positive affirmation and it's a really strong tool. Your mind can control the way you feel, and the way you *feel* is an important factor in determining how you *look*. If you feel well and happy your face will reflect this, but if you are down in the dumps and having a miserable time, your face will soon show this, too. In fact you get the face you deserve by the time you're 40, and one of the keys to looking and feeling younger is being active. The date on a person's birth certificate may not be the best measure of their age.

'GROWING OLD IS SOMETHING YOU DO IF YOU'RE LUCKY'

I don't really believe that age matters or that in this tremendously ageist society that we in the Western world live in, an individual's worth should be judged by the year in which they were born. Older people are sometimes derided and mocked by those who are younger and it's often an attempt at weak one-upmanship. Yes, they may be younger but unfortunately sometimes, they are also overweight, unhappy and living a less-than-healthy lifestyle. Since hopefully today we're all going to live longer, it's essential that we live healthier, more fulfilling lifestyles *whatever* our age, and you're never to old to start this.

One of the main secrets to staying young is staying healthy. I've sometimes had to suppress a smile when some young lady, who has obviously not taken care of herself through diet or exercise, says admiringly, 'Ooh, I hope I look as good as you do when I'm your age!' Although it's intended to be complimentary, it's actually a back-hander.

Even at seventeen I regularly weighed myself – here, on a handy set of butcher's scales.

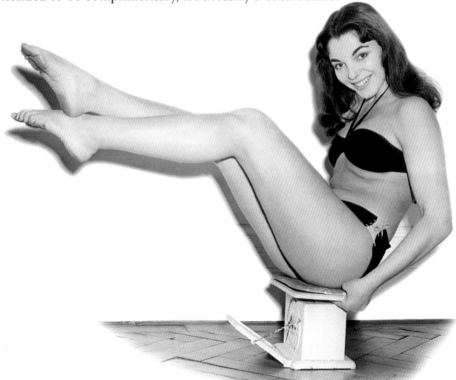

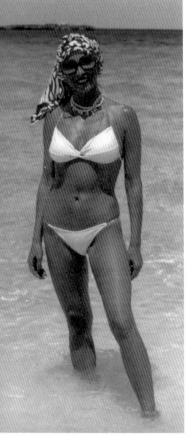

Showing off my tan and my tone in Marbella, circa The Stud, *1979.*

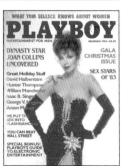

I find the attitude of certain young people – i.e. that being young is to be a superior being – rather pathetic and certainly short-sighted because being young doesn't last, and the less you take care of your inner and outer self, the sooner you will lose that glorious bloom of youth. Let's face it, with today's life expectancy of 80 or more years for women in Britain and the States (around 75 for men), you will be truly young for less than a third of that time and for most of your life you will be officially classed as middle-aged. (I'm not particularly keen on that word either, but I guess it's the only one available.) Youth, as we tend to think of it, actually lasts a terribly short time. Not counting childhood, aged sixteen to 35, is less than twenty years. Not much time, is it?

People started to tell me that I wasn't young any more early on in my career. When, at 25, I told a Hollywood producer my age, he informed me cynically, '25? Honey, that's not young in this town any more.' At 31, when I wanted to start acting again, after having two children, my agent told me: 'Joanie, you're *much* too old to be in the movies any more. Retire, dear, go back to being a housewife and raising the kids.' Needless to say I did *not* take her advice although she put forward a pretty good case for early retirement for actresses.

Then, when I turned 40, I took off most of my clothes and frolicked on a swing in *The Stud*, much to the shock, horror and amazement of all and sundry. But I didn't give a damn. I knew I looked good, very good in fact, and my figure was better than it had ever been, thanks to working out and eating super-healthily.

The Stud became a huge hit and it was because of that movie that I was given the opportunity a few years later to play Alexis Carrington in the hit TV series *Dynasty*. Interestingly enough, one of *Dynasty's* female producers tried hard to prevent me from getting the part because of my age (47). So if that other Hollywood male producer I mentioned thought 25 wasn't young any more in this business, imagine what the other Hollywood producers, who were considering me, along with Sophia Loren and various other actresses, thought? Luckily for me, Mr Aaron Spelling insisted on casting me, so against all the odds I journeyed to Hollywood once more to take on that juicy role and the rest is TV history.

At 49 I posed for a *Playboy* layout and yes, I took off most of my clothes. By this time it had hit me how unbelievably ageist not only Hollywood, but most of the Western world was towards women over 30 and I decided to figuratively thumb my nose at them by proving through my photographs that women 'of a certain age' could still be sexy and alluring. So many older women have thanked me for 'coming out of the closet', as it were and I was given much credit for being the forerunner of the movement who believed older women could still cut it. Today 50 is almost the new 35 and being in your sixties is comparable to how being in your forties was in the 20th century.

When you're older there are so many views you can express that you don't always feel comfortable stating when you're younger. And there have been some great sayings about getting older, too. For example, 'Old age has a great sense of calm and freedom – when the passions relax then hold them. You are freed from the grasp not of one mad master only but of many.' Plato said that, but I don't agree with him – particularly about the passions. The economist Bernard Baruch said, 'Old age is always 15 years older than I am.' That's brilliant. At

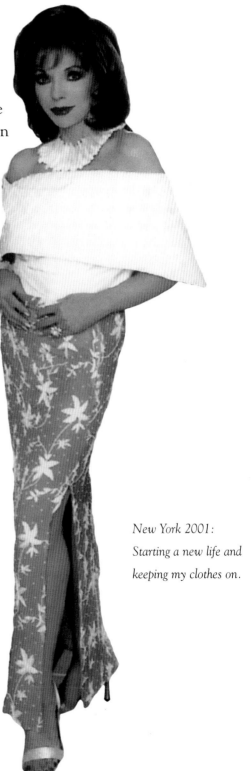

New York 2001:
Starting a new life and
keeping my clothes on.

seventeen I remember thinking 30 was ancient, and at 30, I thought 45 was pretty old, and then at 45, I thought I was in my prime. Think positively. As Groucho Marx said, 'Growing old is something you do if you're lucky'. I think that's great. I mean, so you're getting older? So what's the alternative? No one wants to die, however old they are, and as someone said to the late great Billy Wilder, 'Who wants to be 95?' 'Someone who's 94,' retorted Billy.

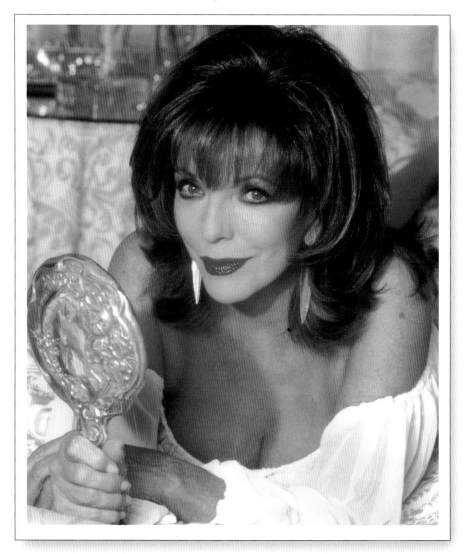

Mirror, mirror in my hand, talk of ageing I can't stand!

After nine years of playing that devious, loveable-hateful bitch Alexis, in haute couture and various stages of deshabillé, I decided to go back to my theatrical roots. I did several more plays, television shows and movies and now in my sixties, I'm happily married to Percy Gibson, a wonderful man who is more than three decades younger than me. To him, it doesn't matter a jot how old I am, and it doesn't matter to me either. We are extremely happy together and astonishingly compatible in every way. He loves me not only for the way I look but also for my tremendous enthusiasm, energy and *joie de vivre*, which I was lucky enough to be born with and intend to keep for as long as I can. When people ask me, *sotto voce* in surprise, 'So what about the age difference between you and Percy?' I usually shrug, smile and quip, 'So, if he dies, he dies.'

Actually, it amazes me that the older woman–younger man relationship comes in for so much criticism. More and more bright, intelligent and attractive women are marrying and having relationships with men who are ten, twenty and even 30 years their junior. Many of them say they've never been happier and I have to say, I agree.

So how *do* you stave off the ageing process? In this chapter I shall attempt to impart the advice, wisdom and knowledge I've gathered and studied pretty much since I was a teenager when I first started out in this business. From the moment we are born our skin starts to age, as does our hair, bones and teeth – everything. Just look at the skin of a newborn and that of a ten-year-old, then compare the ten-year-old's complexion with that of a 25-year-old and you see the difference.

My mother, Elsa Bessant Collins, was really beautiful. Blonde and blue-eyed, she had the pale delicate skin that goes with the territory and she took great care of it, too. I always remember her using a product called Glymiel Jelly on her hands and knees, and she tried to get me to use it but it was so thick and gloopy that I wasn't tempted. Mummie and her eight sisters had excellent skin, as did my father's two sisters and my paternal grandmother Hettie, and they had masses of paints and potions on their dressing tables. Fascinated, I used to watch as they anointed themselves and they really seemed to get pleasure out of the feminine arts of adornment.

Women weren't ashamed to enjoy pampering themselves with make-up, perfume and hairdos then. And it worked. Looking at pictures of my family and their friends, they all seemed groomed and glamorous. But women seemed to age much earlier then than they do now, perhaps because they were not so well nourished as today's women. If you look at a photograph of a 25-year-old in the forties or fifties, she'll look 35.

Although the life span for humans may be more than 100 years, life expectancy is not anticipated to rise much above 85 today, even if cures are found for cancer and heart disease. Progressive natural loss of organ functioning puts a biological limit of about 85 years on life expectancy. Eliminating heart disease could add three years, and conquering cancer would, on average, add two.

It's important to distinguish between life *span* and life *expectancy*. Life span is characteristic of a species – two or three years for mice, 45 years for chimpanzees and 110 to 120 for humans, although there have been reports of humans living even longer, but most scientists don't believe them. A 50-year-old woman today has a life expectancy of 85 and if you're younger than 50 you could hit 90.

Life expectancy for a species is based on projections of how long 50% of a group will survive. Until about 1850, life expectancy for humans ranged between 30 and 40 years. Then, in 1900, a person born in a developed country could expect to live an average of 50 years. By 1946, life expectancy had risen to 67, and today it averages out at about 74.

While most people credit medical advances since the middle of the 19th century, evidence indicates that improvements in transportation (enabling more intermarriage and strengthening of the gene pool), nutrition, sanitation, education and housing are largely responsible for the dramatic increase in life expectancy.

SLOWING THE CLOCK

For centuries man (and woman) has searched for the elusive fountain of youth. Up to a point it *can* be achieved and I'm going to show you some ways in which you can at least slow the clock. First of all, it's important to understand that ageing and disease are two different things. Ageing is the mysterious process that inevitably leads to death, while disease can be the result of individual lifestyle. It seems logical therefore that we can slow down the ageing process by staying healthy and thus often prevent degenerative diseases.

Certainly, at 35 or 40 you're not going to have the dewy cheeks of a 20-year-old, but through discipline and knowledge you *can* keep that 20-year-old skin and body looking as good as possible for years to come, and it's *never too late to start*. No one says it's easy, however. Scientists today increasingly report that debilitation in middle and old age is mainly caused by improper nourishment, poor eating habits and lack of exercise. There are few short cuts to ageing well and if you want to get the best out of life after middle age, you should start working towards that goal from a relatively young age.

However, if you're not in the first flush of youth don't despair. Even 60- and 70-year-olds can see a huge improvement through watching their diet carefully and exercising regularly. You've got to use it or lose it. Unless it's taken care of, nothing will work properly or wear well if it's not used and this is particularly true of the human body. Try not speaking for a few days when you've had a sore throat. When you next attempt conversation, you will be hard-pressed to make your tongue and vocal chords do what they were used to doing and the longer you don't talk, the longer it will take to get back to normal.

It's the same with any part of your body. If you rarely walk, your legs will become weaker and if you loll around like a couch spud, they'll atrophy. And if you don't do some sort of exercise, which involves using every part of your body, at least two or, ideally, three times a week, you will eventually become lethargic and feeble. Then you will lose bone density, the flexibility of your joints and muscles will start to go and after a certain age, you will almost certainly begin to shrink. If you were athletic as a teenager and you continue to be so, you could still be strong and healthy well into your seventies or eighties. At the age of 70 some swimmers can still do their laps or even swim the Channel almost as well as when they were in their twenties. This goes for runners and dancers, too. I have a friend in her seventies, Gillian Lynne, the famous choreographer of *Cats*, among many other shows, whose body hasn't changed one iota since she was twenty. She says the main reason for this is that she has never stopped doing her daily *barré* exercises and she works with dancers a third of her age.

Now let's get to grips with this ageing business to see what can be done about it. If we can't stop the clock, let us at least try to slow it down. Ageing is a horrible word, which is all too often used in the most derogatory way by the media – 'wrinkly rocker', 'ageing actress', etc. It's almost as though it's used to denote total uselessness in a person. You can't help getting older, but you *can* help yourself from becoming old and infirm, in mind as well as body. In particular you should *stop* thinking that getting older bars you from the joys and benefits of youthful pursuits, such as sports or socialising. In the past 50 years the number of people over 60, many of whom are living extremely productive, happy lives, has practically doubled. The later years can be active and rewarding, and getting sick isn't an inevitable part of getting older. Research on both sides of the Atlantic indicates that self-healing can be achieved through appropriate choices in diet and exercise. With a rapidly ageing and increasingly sedentary population in the western world (the number of people aged 60 and over is projected to increase from 12 million in 2002 to 18.6 million in 2031).

Some of the latest styles in the fashion magazines send the author into paroxysms of amusement.

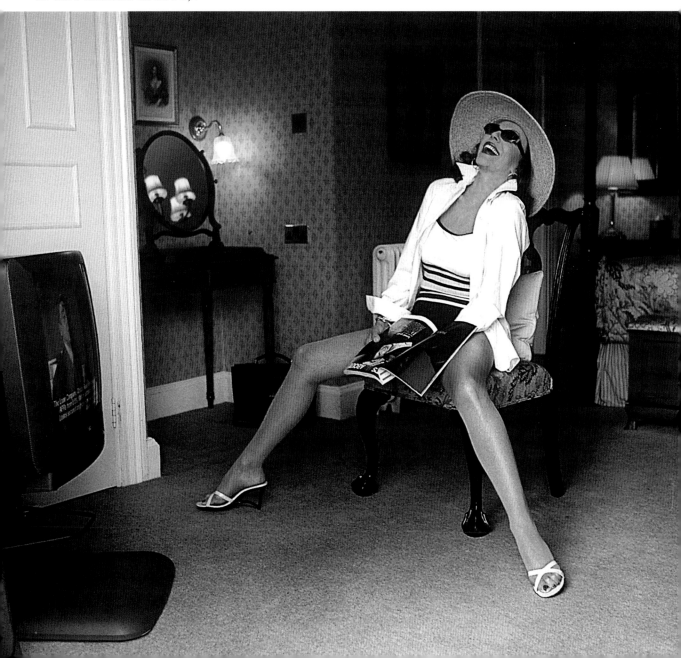

BEATING THE CLOCK

Osteoporosis and arthritis were once considered an old lady's lot. Lucky enough to live to a ripe old age, she would inevitably become so crippled and disabled that she would be condemned to a life of pain and unable to take care of herself. Today, by the age of 50 the average woman has lost up to one third of her bone mass. Sadly, osteoporosis will affect one woman in two in later life and in some families the risk is even greater. It's an insidious disease that creeps up over the years. Bones slowly lose their tissue and become weaker and more brittle until they eventually waste away. Until fractures occur, this often goes unnoticed, by which time it may be too late to do anything about it. Although everyone suffers from osteoporosis to some degree, people who smoke and drink excessively, have more than six cups of coffee a day, who hardly ever exercise and have small bones may be more prone to it and can start to suffer earlier.

Another natural stage in life is the onset of the menopause. In Britain half a million women go through the menopause every year. About a third of these suffer from exceedingly uncomfortable symptoms, including night sweats and hot flushes. Menopause and childbirth are the highest contributory factors to the advancement of osteoporosis, which is why it's important to include plenty of calcium and iron in your diet in the form of dairy products (alternatively fortified soya milk and soya products such as tofu), green leafy vegetables, fish and dried fruits.

Once they reach 50, many women believe their productive lives to be over. When they look in the mirror they see a body they think is either too fat or too scrawny, skin that has lost its lustre and dull or greying hair. But there are plenty of things you can do to combat this. Hormone Replacement Therapy (HRT) – or Estrogen Replacement Therapy (ERT) as it's known in the States – is a controversial subject, but I believe it to be the greatest gift to older women, as significant in its way as the contraceptive pill is to those of childbearing age. Taken in the correct dosage HRT can help bypass many of the problems of menopause. It can help you retain your zest for life and radically slow down the ageing process and help in the battle against osteoporosis. It can also improve your sex life (see page 165).

In my opinion, HRT is the miracle drug. Although many doctors still pooh pooh or condemn it completely, it can prevent brittle bones, increase energy levels, help protect the body from strokes and heart attacks, improve memory and concentration levels, and make dull skin glow again. As I have experienced myself, HRT can keep your bones as strong as they ever were. When I was performing in a play recently I had two bad falls backstage. Once, while running down some steps, I slipped and fell, taking my entire body weight on both knees. The other time I managed to fall up the steps, landing hard on my wrists and elbows. Because I have strong bones I suffered nothing more serious than minor bruising and slight discomfort. However, the incidence of brittle bone disease in older women is truly terrifying. For some, a simple fall can mean several bones, particularly wrists and hips, are broken and they may never heal properly again. Other HRT supporters in the public eye include the Iron Lady herself, Baroness Margaret Thatcher, actress Cheryl Ladd and supermodel Lauren Hutton.

Among the other great benefits of HRT are that it replaces vitality and provides a renewed zest for life that the menopause can take away. Many women in their sixties and seventies on HRT have begun lucrative second careers, written their first novel, taken up painting, given talks to women's groups and even learnt to fly.

However, if HRT doesn't agree with you – which unfortunately, is the case for some women – there are other ways to prevent osteoporosis and to help with some of the less welcome effects of menopause. A diet rich in calcium and vitamin D or a supplement, and regular weight-bearing exercise, like walking or dancing, will help to keep bones healthy. Many women swear by red clover, and linseed oil and vitamin E are both good for dry skin: all are available as supplements.

HRT isn't a magic pill that will turn you into a young girl again but it can most certainly improve the quality of your life in many ways. So run, don't walk to your nearest GP (physician). If he turns out to be one of the non-believers, find a doctor who is a believer. But, and I cannot stress this enough, HRT *must* be prescribed in the correct dosage for you and that usually starts with the minimum amount. Also, although research is at the time of going to press inconclusive, there are reports of an increased susceptibility to breast cancer. So if you do decide to take it, it's essential to have a yearly mammogram just to play it safe. My doctor has assured me that the benefits far outweigh the risks but before you make up your mind depending on your own circumstances, seek professional medical advice.

PRIME TIME

Once the kids have flown the nest (or you've retired), it's time to achieve your private ambitions, and even if these are not so ambitious as piloting planes or writing bestsellers, there's a whole world of things to do and achieve out there. Don't write yourself off simply because you've had a milestone birthday that ends in a nought. This may have been understandable at the beginning of the last century when the sands of time were definitely running out for a woman who reached 40, but today there are decades ahead when you could do so many things. Write, paint, sculpt, learn the piano, take up dancing, whether it's the tango or line dancing, start a university or college course, fall in love all over again – the possibilities are limitless.

Now is the time to be a little selfish. Many of today's older women have devoted their lives to a man, perhaps children or maybe to caring for elderly parents, so it's fine, when the big five or six-0 hits, to take some time for yourself, to pamper yourself in every way. You've sure earned it, girl. After all, if you won't do it, who's going to do it for you?

I believe that to help keep bones strong and healthy in later life, HRT is essential. To this end, I also recommend you take the following:

A daily dose of Vitamin E capsules.

A fish supplement, such as Maxepa or cod-liver oil.

Antioxidant vitamins to prevent the free radicals, which cause ageing.

Calcium pills.

Vitamin A – which is a great healer – and Vitamin D to promote absorption of calcium into the bones.

MSM (Methyl Sulphonyl/Sulfonyl Methane). Essential for people over 50 with incipient arthritis or osteoporosis.

Plenty of the following foods: sardines in olive oil and other fatty fish such as tuna, smoked salmon and haddock; milk, cheese and eggs (but don't overdo the dairy – too much builds up cholesterol). To maintain healthy bones, it's as essential for older women as it is for infants and young children to get that calcium.

Beta-carotene. After Vitamins E and C, it's the most powerful antioxidant. Not only does it fight free radicals, it also slows down and can prevent skin cancer. To boost your intake, eat as much as you can of the following: beetroot, broccoli, spinach, tomatoes, papaya, watercress, tomato sauce, cantaloupe, plus at least one 85g (3oz) serving of green, red or yellow vegetables a day.

By the way, there is a difference between osteoporosis and osteoarthritis. The latter is a form of arthritis in which the cartilage of the joint and bone are worn away, due to an injury or wear and tear on the joints, often caused by sports injuries. My father suffered badly from osteoarthritis in both his hands. I've inherited it slightly – luckily only in my thumbs – but I'm able to keep it under control. When I learnt that certain kinds of arthritis were hereditary, I started to take precautions. I take several Vitamin E tablets a day plus Maxepa, a fish oil supplement, and MSM, a rich source of organic sulphur. In addition to this, I sometimes wear a copper bracelet on my wrist and if my thumbs start to hurt, I occasionally take a teaspoon of cider vinegar with honey in hot water. Another new method for treating arthritis is magnets. I have a set of armbands with small magnets inside and although no one knows why and how they work, they ease the pain. I first discovered them at an American sports injuries clinic and although I was dubious, they *really* help.

FIGHT FREE RADICALS

Some of the outward signs of ageing – wrinkles, liver spots, lack of elasticity in the skin – are caused by disruption of the internal workings of the cells and also certain cellular proteins, such as collagen, between the cells. The reason for this is oxidisation, a cell-damaging process caused by molecular fragments known as free radicals. Antioxidants help to neutralise them and the best way to get them is through your diet. Here's a list of foods that will help combat this insidious enemy. Make sure you eat at least one or two portions each day. The best of the best are:
• Apricots, broccoli, cantaloupes, carrots, dark leafy vegetables, spinach, mangos, peaches, pumpkins and sweet potatoes.
Also beneficial are:
• Asparagus, Brussels sprouts, green beans, peas, tomatoes and watermelon.

So what are these free radicals that contribute so much to the ageing process? They are tiny, highly reactive molecules created during normal metabolism and from our polluted world. They can inflict the kind of cellular damage that leads to heart disease, cancer, brain disorders and other degenerative diseases including ageing. And how can they hurt us? In their molecular structure, free radicals are unbalanced. They have an odd number of electrons in their outermost molecular ring and to be 'satisfied' they either have to steal an electron, or give one up. This means forcibly snatching one from a nearby cell, or shooting an electron into a cell. While this satisfies the free radical, it also begins the destruction of the other cell and starts off a chain reaction. Each cell, in turn, gains or loses an unwanted electron. It's the same kind of reaction that occurs when butter becomes rancid. Can you imagine what happens to you when the fat in your body turns rancid? Chemical changes inside living cells can cause genetic mutation, alter the structure of important proteins, disable fatty molecules, and more. If the damage accumulates faster than the body repairs it, disease and premature ageing can be the result. To survive, a cell needs a variety of defence mechanisms that will destroy the free radicals before they do any damage.

Auctioning off these Teletubbies at a charity in aid of breast cancer. (London, 1998).

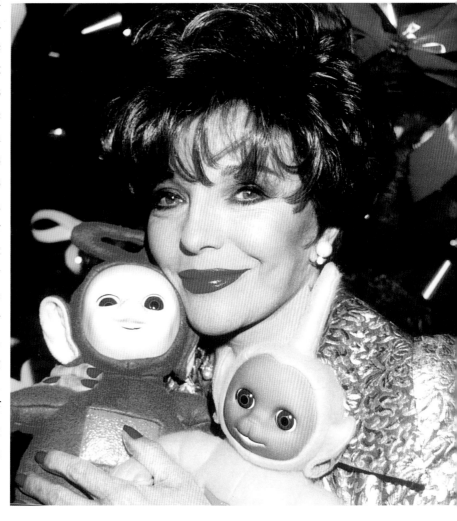

Unfortunately, free radical damage to certain types of cells is irreversible. It's a fact, however, that although 98 per cent of free radicals is burned up for energy, unfortunately that leaves 2 per cent available for non-productive harmful activity. Three types of cells – heart, muscle and nerve cells, which include brain cells and certain sensor cells of the immune system – *cannot* be replaced. To ensure a long and healthy life, damage to these cells must be prevented. After years of free radical assault, millions of cells are lost from major organs such as the lungs, kidneys, liver and brain. Cell loss is a major cause of ageing and free radicals have been linked to a wide range of conditions associated with it. They pose a greater problem in later life because as you get older, the body's ability to neutralise free radicals and repair the damage they cause goes into decline. As free radicals are a by-product of normal metabolic processes, you probably produce more when you are younger and more metabolically active. Their extremely reactive nature means they have considerable potential for oxidative cell damage, including damage to cell integrity, harmful changes to capillaries and damage to the collagen and elastin in skin.

But diet alone cannot protect you and that's why vitamin supplements are *essential*. Vitamin E is the number one for counteracting the effects of oxidation. I call it the magic vitamin after Vitamin C. It has many other benefits. Combined with Vitamin C, researchers have discovered that Vitamin E can help counteract cataract formation, which is caused by the oxidation of eye lenses. Vitamin E also delays the progress and reduces the severity of Parkinson's Disease. It also boosts the immune system (the body's defence against infectious diseases). Beta-carotene, too, can help combat free radicals.

In fact, the power of vitamins should never be underestimated. Some time ago now *The New York Times* reported provocative new evidence from researchers, indicating that 'vitamins influence the health and vibrancy of nearly every organ, and that these enigmatic chemicals may help forestall or even reverse many diseases of ageing'.

I for one am not too keen on taking drugs and pills. Sure, they can be used to ease the symptoms of diabetes and heart disease, but I don't want to get sick in the first place so I take preventative measures through eating good food and exercising. I can't stress the importance of this enough and most scientists do now believe that exercise and proper nutrition can help to stave off everything from heart disease to diabetes, osteoporosis and ageing.

Whatever you do, you can't prevent the inevitable natural changes that occur with getting older – skin, bones, muscles, teeth, hair, eyes, heart, lungs, over time these all change and to function properly, the body needs a constant and balanced amount of the right nutrients and vitamins.

Some gerontologists believe ageing results from the accumulated damage done to cells throughout the years, usually caused by toxicity in the environment, pollution and food preservatives. Others believe genetics determines ageing – if your parents looked good for their age, the chances are that you will, too. This is true, but only up to a point so you've still got to take care of yourself. Anyway, doesn't a not-so attractive person who has aged well look better than an attractive one who hasn't paid attention to this?

OBESITY IS SPREADING (LITERALLY)

One of the major health problems the Western world faces today is obesity. Except in extremely rare genetic cases, obesity is basically caused by eating too much and not exercising enough. So plump children become fat teenagers, who will then become obese adults, who will almost certainly contract life-threatening diseases such as diabetes and strokes. In America the number of obese adults has doubled in the past ten years, and the number of grossly obese people (overweight by 44 kilos/98 pounds or more) has grown even more. One in 80 American men and one in 200 women now weighs more than 133 kilos/294 pounds, a leap of 50 per cent in four years. A growing number of people over the age of 40 are now developing late-onset (or Type 2) diabetes, but have you noticed that there are very few obese 70-year-olds? Sadly, they don't live that long.

All the excuses you hear from overweight people – that it's genetic or glandular – are often wishful thinking, I'm afraid. The reason why fat is stored in the body is because it's not used for the day-to-day energy the body needs to function. To put it bluntly, by eating too much they are digging their own graves with their teeth. Without doubt, obesity is one of the most dangerous contributors to ageing and the precursor of many deadly diseases. Both here and in the States, doctors predict that obesity will be *the* major health crisis of the next generation. The National Association to Advance Fat Acceptance (NAAFA) has thrived since 1972. Their arguments are that there's no such thing as permanent weight loss and their members are fat because of genetics, not because they eat too much. With respect, these arguments are much too weak to promote the acceptance of obesity and certainly, it's as wrong to discriminate against the obese as it is to discriminate against any other group. But to condone obesity is to ignore the fact that overweight people face very serious health risks in later life and this is being proven all the time. Not only this, but being overweight also prevents people from making the most of life. They tend to have less energy and feel tired; they may also suffer from poor self-image and it's much harder to get around.

During food rationing in the First World War there was a huge reduction in the obesity of the citizens of Europe and the States. With that came a reduction in the obesity-related diseases of diabetes and hypertension. Doesn't that tell you something about our diets today? In the thirties experiments were conducted on laboratory rats at

Cornell University. One group was fed as much as they liked for 24 hours a day while another was calorie-controlled and given just enough to live on. When they all finally died, it was found that the group who grazed all day lived for an average of 483 days, while the calorie-controlled rats survived for an astonishing 900 days (almost twice as long). Those scientists also discovered that the calorie-controlled rats acted younger, looked younger and by the physiological standards of ageing actually *were* younger. Now it has been ultimately proved that eating less extends your life span. But, and it's a big but (and I'm sure you don't want one of those!), if you eat less you *must* make sure that what you eat is nutritionally sound and enriched with the correct amounts of vitamins and minerals.

In 1970 only 4 per cent of American children aged six to twelve were overweight. Today, that number is over 15 per cent. Who knows what it will be in the next decade? It's a terrifying thought. We live in the fast-food era where many kids and adults eat fatty hamburgers or hot dogs or rich takeaways, pre-packaged and packed with additives, or frozen food that just needs to be reheated, for most meals. Although many people say they don't have time to cook, healthy stir-fries and pasta with tomato sauce do not take that long to prepare.

Junk food is just that – *junk*. Although I rarely ate hamburgers, I stopped eating them altogether when I saw a picture of a woman who had taken a bite out of one in a burger joint and found she had bitten into a mouse! Ugh! If I ever had a reason to stop, that was it. Nevertheless, the fast-food industry is a multibillion dollar business and I'm sure they must put something addictive in those burgers for everyone to crave them so much and so often. One of the most chilling statistics I discovered when writing this book was that a third of all human cancers are directly related to diet. Another recent report by Britain's Office for National Statistics confirmed that the number of diabetics in Britain could double by 2020, largely due to the British dislike of healthy food, and some scientists have linked this to bad eating habits, lack of exercise and obesity. But there is some positive news. In a move designed to protect companies from the kind of lawsuits brought against the tobacco industry, junk food companies in the States are to warn consumers that eating too much of their products could fatten them up. The project, which is backed by the International Food Information Council Foundation, could lead to packaged foods such as chocolate cookies and crisps (chips) having similar warnings.

Sugary fizzy drinks are also bad for your body. They are loaded with sodium, artificial additives and colourings, and the bubbles can make you extremely bloated. I never drink sodas and I might have a couple of Coca Colas a year, but *never* Diet Coke as I believe the ingredients in it, particularly the artificial sweetener and aspartame are bad for you. And I've been told they can make you depressed or feel tired. I've never allowed my own children to drink fizzy or so-called energy drinks. I always gave them natural fruit drinks.

So, for super-youth, here is my list of super foods to help halt the onset of the disease and ageing process:

✔ Chicken – white meat only, not the skin
✔ Lean beef (but only occasionally)
✔ Salmon and mackerel
✔ Tuna, trout, haddock and cod
✔ Skimmed or low-fat milk
✔ Non-processed cheese
✔ Low-fat yoghurt
✔ Skimmed mozzarella cheese
✔ Leafy green vegetables especially broccoli
✔ Fresh vegetables
✔ Fresh fruit and juices, but not from a can

- ✓ Whole grains
- ✓ Brown rice
- ✓ Wholemeal (whole-wheat) flour
- ✓ Couscous
- ✓ Pinto, haricot (navy) and kidney beans
- ✓ Olive oil
- ✓ Sunflower oil
- ✓ Peanut oil
- ✓ Safflower oil
- ✓ Hummus
- ✓ Taramasalata
- ✓ Anchovies (canned or fresh)
- ✓ Sardines in olive oil
- ✓ Nuts (particularly almonds which are reputed to have cancer-preventing qualities)
- ✓ Wine (in moderation). Studies of 1,555 New Yorkers by scientists at the University of Buffalo (USA) prove that people who drink wine, particularly white wine, have healthier lungs than those who drink beer or spirits. Red wine, too, brings down cholesterol as it thins the blood.
- ✓ Chocolate (also in moderation)
- ✓ Still mineral water. The British Dietetic Association guidelines state that the average adult should consume 2.5 litres (4½ pints) a day. Of this 1.8 litres (3 pints) must be obtained directly from water (the equivalent of 6–7 glasses per day). To avoid dehydration, intake should be increased in hot weather and during as well as after physical activity.

THE FOUNTAIN OF YOUTH

Juan Ponce de Leon (1474–1521) was a Spanish explorer and conquistador who was obsessed with tales of the Fountain of Youth, a mythical fountain which was reputed to flow with water that cured illness and granted the drinker eternal youth. As he searched for it, he became the first European to explore Puerto Rico, Florida, the Florida Keys and parts of Mexico. But Ponce de Leon never found the Fountain of Youth because it's *within* us all. You've just got to work to find it, so here are my rules for the *real* Fountain of Youth:

✓ A positive attitude

✓ Staying healthy, which means eating healthily with optimum nutrition

✓ Regular exercise (at least three times per week for 40 minutes)

✓ Relaxation through avoidance of stress wherever possible

✓ Love, whether with a partner, child, pet or friends.

And here is my list of No No's or destructive elements:

✗ White bread

✗ White sugar

✗ Doughnuts and cookies, which are drenched in fat and sugar

✗ Hamburgers

✗ Processed meats

✗ Processed cheese

✗ Smoked meats (except smoked salmon in small quantities)

✗ Rancid fat and stale food of any kind

✗ Bar-b-cued meat

✗ Burnt toast

✗ Pizza

✗ Salt and pepper

✗ Saturated fat and fried foods

✗ Food that's heavily spiced

✗ Store-bought cakes

✗ Butter (unless in moderation)

✗ Alcohol

✗ Tap water.

Just another morning waiting for breakfast in bed!

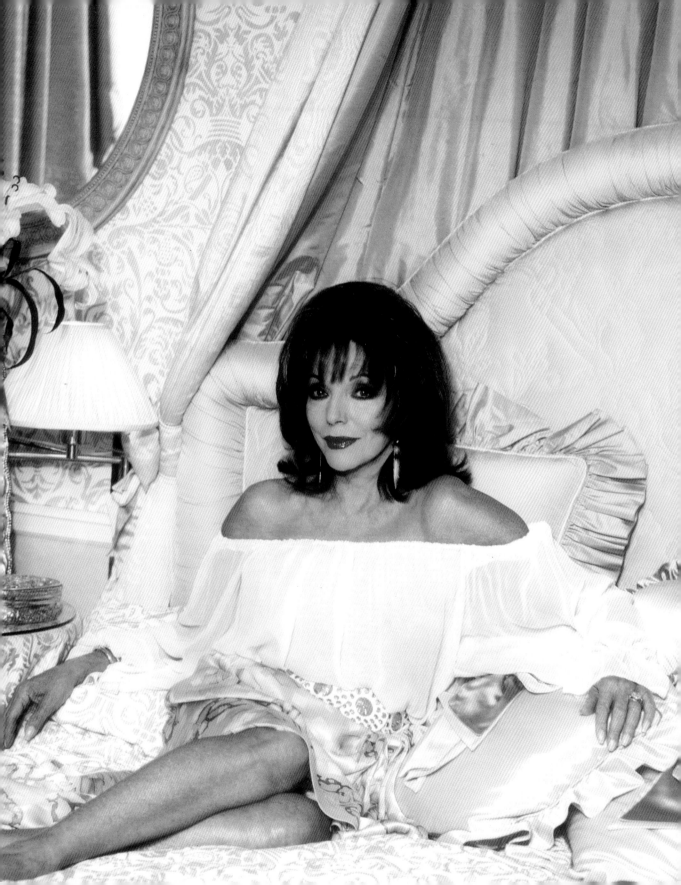

No diets please

Chapter 2

Eating right for life

Without a doubt the most important thing you can do to maintain maximum health, vitality and youthfulness is to eat properly and by this I *don't* mean dieting. Dieting seldom, if ever, works and when it does, it's relatively short-term. Yes, you certainly can lose ten to twenty pounds with a crash diet, such as the Banana-and-Milk or the Carrot-and-Cottage-Cheese, or the million other diets that are around. But ultimately, unless you change your way of eating and *what* you eat, the pounds will pile back on again, and probably more of them.

Did you know that the more you eat and the *more frequently* you eat, the more you will stretch your stomach which therefore needs even more food to feel full? So, if you've been stuffing yourself, stop now because it's possible to feel satisfied without eating until you burst. One of the reasons so many of us are overweight is because the amount of food one is given in restaurants (or any other eating establishments these days) is obscene. When I was growing up, no one was given an enormous plate overflowing with food. The fact that the average person today is at least twenty to thirty pounds heavier than their peers from the fifties and sixties says it all. As for the combinations of food served they simply are appalling. In some restaurants in the States 'Surf & Turf', consisting of a huge chunk of red meat and a whole lobster tail drenched in butter, plus all the trimmings like fries and coleslaw (full of sugar) is extremely popular. Imagine how harmful this is not only for your digestion but also your cholesterol levels. But people go on eating it and just get bigger and bigger and more and more unhealthy.

The average hamburger will also contain white bread, processed meat (using most of the animal parts), cheese, ketchup (catsup), mayonnaise and French fries. It contains about 1,500 calories which is more than half of what a grown man should eat a day. Add to that a sweet fizzy drink and ice cream with all the trimmings and one meal puts you far over the edge of the daily recommended calorific intake. It's also a nutritional nightmare.

In my days as a TV social worker I fed the starving in the soup kitchen. (Star Trek, circa 1960s.)

Recently I went into a pub for lunch and ordered a simple salad. Here's what I got on my plate: celery, rice, nut and raisin mush, cucumber, strawberries, pasta shells, pears in cream, lettuce, orange slices, raspberries, coleslaw and grapes. No wonder Britain is following close behind the States in the obesity stakes. When I only ate about a quarter, I was asked if everything was all right.

Overeating is undoubtedly one of the main causes of disease and premature ageing. In a study of centenarians, scientists discovered that there's no such thing as an obese centenarian – because a very fat person seldom lives that long. Impressive advances have been made through research into inexpensive diet, exercise and lifestyle changes attainable by virtually anybody at any age, the theory being that the body has the potential for regeneration that can be hampered or exploited by everyday habits. As Benjamin Franklin

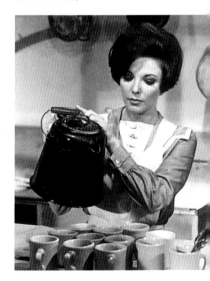

said, 'To lengthen the life, lessen the meals.' Or take another truism from Dr Paavo Airola, 'A man's belt length determines his life length. The longer the belt, the shorter the life.' It's important to look after your body when you're relatively young to pave the way for a healthier middle and older life.

I shudder whenever I see advertisements for the 'Fat Boy' breakfasts: 'All you can eat for $1.99' – fried eggs, bacon, sausages, hash brown potatoes, pancakes and maple syrup. It's a cholesterol bomb and a potential crippler.

So here are some of my ideas for the healthiest and most beneficial style of eating. Try them for a week and not only will you have lost weight, you will also feel more energetic, less sluggish and ready to *live*!

First of all, don't ever eat or shop for food when you're hungry. Temptation is all around you in the supermarket.

Eat three meals a day only. Try not to graze. You're not a cow!

If you *must* eat between meals, choose one of the following:

• One apple (70 calories)
• One peach (85 calories)
• Half a can of sardines in oil (80 calories)
• Three crackers (150 calories)
• Half a banana (70 calories)
• A small packet of crisps (chips) (140 calories)
• A glass of wine (80 calories)
• 50g (2oz) mozzarella (170 calories)
• Five sticks of broccoli (50 calories)
• One Ryvita or crispbread (15 calories) with either one teaspoon of Marmite (50 calories) or cream cheese (20 calories)
• One hard-boiled egg (75 calories)
• Half a KitKat if you're desperate for chocolate. Can you believe it's only 110 calories?

At a restaurant, do not finish everything on your plate. I try to eat only two-thirds of what I am served.

Avoid drinking alcohol during meals. (I'm afraid I cheat as I love a glass of wine with dinner.)

Drink a large glass of still water before eating – it fills your stomach so you'll eat less.

Don't drink alcohol until 20 minutes after you have finished eating.

Eliminate or cut down on salt and pepper.

Cut out booze, or just have one glass of wine a day.

Don't drink soft or fizzy drinks or sugary squash-type juices and reduce your intake of coffee and tea. (I'm hopeless at this. I *have* to have my coffee in the morning. For extra calcium, I drink 50ml (2fl oz, ¼ cup) milk throughout the day with my coffee.) Try not to have more than three cups of tea or coffee a day, or try herbal or fruit teas.

Don't eat anything made from refined white flour or white sugar. That means cakes, biscuits (cookies), sweets (candies), etc. – all the goodies, unfortunately.

And now for a few recipes.

ON WAKING UP
• A large glass of bottled water (tap water is not good for you – I don't drink it because I'm not keen on recycled urine, hormones and antibiotics). If you wish, add a squeeze of fresh lemon, lime, grapefruit or orange.

BREAKFAST
• Half a bowl of chopped fresh fruit such as bananas, apples, oranges, grapes and berries.

• A 100g (4oz) carton of low-fat yoghurt and one slice of wholemeal (whole-wheat) toast with low-fat butter or butter substitute (I highly recommend 'I Can't Believe It's Not Butter') and/or low-sugar jam.

———— Or ————

• A small bowl of oatmeal with four or five prunes or figs and a sprinkling of raisins.
• One cup of herbal tea sweetened with honey, if needed. (I cheat and have coffee!)

———— Or ————

One freshly squeezed orange, apple or pear juice.

LUNCH

• A bowl of freshly prepared vegetable soup with one slice of wholemeal (whole-wheat), sour dough or rye bread, and low-fat or butter substitute. One or two small slices of natural Cheddar or brie (not processed cheese).

———— Or ————

• A large bowl of fresh vegetable salad including tomatoes, avocados, lamb's lettuce (mâche), corn salad, carrots, rocket (arugula), beetroot (beets) and onions (important for good health). Raw garlic, too (just don't breathe on too many people). A light dressing of lemon juice (or cider vinegar) and olive oil and a little sea-salt. One hard-boiled (hard-cooked) egg.

———— Or ————

• One can of sardines in pure olive oil, two large tomatoes (sliced) and a salad of raw spinach with a light dressing.

———— Or ————

• A two-egg omelette (with only the yolk of one), herbs and a small salad of lettuce, lamb's lettuce (mâche), cucumber and grated carrots.

———— Or ————

• Half an avocado stuffed with a large tablespoon of lightly curried white turkey meat mixed with one teaspoon of low-fat mayonnaise, one teaspoon of sweetcorn and 50g (2oz, ½ cup) of finely chopped cucumber. You can also substitute canned tuna for the turkey meat.

———— *Or* ————

• 85g (3oz) of cold salmon in a light dill sauce and sliced cucumber with a touch of vinegar.

———— *Or* ————

• 250ml (8fl oz, 1 cup) of mushroom and barley soup, 175g (6oz, 1 cup) of steamed cabbage and a small vegetable salad.

DINNER

• 250ml (8fl oz, 1 cup) of onion soup, 85g (3oz) lean lamb chop, 150g (5oz, 1 cup) of string beans and a large green salad.

———— *Or* ————

• One steamed artichoke, 100g (4oz) baked flounder (or cod or sea bass) and a large vegetable salad.

———— *Or* ————

• 100g (4oz) baked chicken breast (skinned) plus 150g (5oz, 1 cup) of carrots stir-fried with ginger and about 225g (8oz, 2 cups) of steamed okra, zucchini and cauliflower.

———— *Or* ————

• Half an avocado and watercress salad. Six spears of asparagus and 225g (8oz, 1 cup) of steamed yellow squash.

———— *Or* ————

• 225g (8oz, 2 cups) of curried chicken and vegetables and 225g (8oz, 2 cups) of cucumber and vegetable salad.

———— *Or* ————

• 100g (4oz) tuna fish and 175g (6oz, 1 cup) of steamed spinach salad.

———— *Or* ————

• Six spears of asparagus, 100g (4oz) baked sole, 150g (5oz, 1 cup) of brown rice and a large vegetable salad.

If you *must* have dessert, then make it half a low-fat yoghurt or one scoop of sorbet. I don't think eating fruit after meals is terribly good for you. It sits on top of the food eaten and doesn't pass through you. I only eat fruit in the morning.

FIGHT THOSE HUNGER PANGS

Drinking a few glasses of water is a proven way to fill up your stomach and that hunger-free feeling can last an hour or even longer. I know the portions I've listed above sound paltry and as though you're denying yourself, but just remember that you're not – you are just going back to eating the healthy sensible portions your body requires. You may feel hungry in the first week but as time goes on, your body will be satisfied with the normal calorific intake and the yearnings (because that's what they are) will subside. It isn't easy, it takes resolve, strength of mind and willpower, but it's worth it. Sensible eating could help you to live for twenty years longer. It might even save your life.

Billions of pounds a year are wasted on weight-loss pills, potions and so-called magic liquid diets, most of which don't work in the long run. I would never go on one of these diets. Remember when Oprah Winfrey lost 80 pounds on a liquid diet and was on the cover of *Vogue*, looking gorgeous? Yes, it was a miracle but unfortunately it didn't last. As soon as Oprah started eating solid foods again, her weight went up and up. Two years later she was heavier than she had been before and not at all happy about this, *despite* having her own specialist live-in chef and a personal trainer.

Balzac once said, 'There is no such thing as great talent without great willpower' and someone who lost a great deal of weight and did it the right way, proving she *does* have the willpower, is my friend Liza Minelli. A year ago, Liza was a mess, and she admits it. She was 100 pounds overweight, bloated, sick and almost unable to walk.

Today, with the help of her new husband, David Gest, she has lost nearly all that weight, and at the age of 56 is healthy, happy and working on stage better than ever before. Recently Percy and I saw her perform in *Liza's Back* at the Albert Hall in London. She looked and *was* stunning. At dinner afterwards Liza eschewed the risotto we all had and opted for a salad of lettuce and tomatoes.

Then, for her 'fish and chips' main course, she ate the fish and some (but not all) of the potatoes. She didn't deny herself – she just didn't stuff herself. Well done, Liza! Now she looks fabulous, and it's all down to healthy eating, moderation, motivation and *discipline*.

HOW I MAINTAIN MY WEIGHT

Unfortunately, many people don't have the willpower to stop indulging in the pizzas, fried chicken and mashed potatoes everyone loves. Who doesn't love pizza and mashed potatoes? I know I do, and I

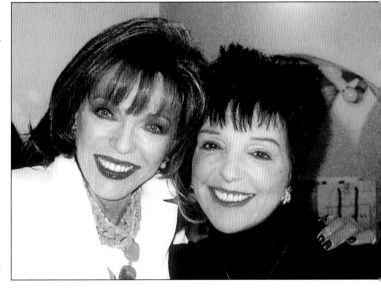

Life is a cabaret again for Liza Minelli. Backstage at the Albert Hall with Liza, who is looking better than ever and is consequently happier than ever, too. (London, 2002)

won't deny myself, but never more than once or twice a month and then I'll only eat less than half a portion.

Because I know just how easy it is to put on weight and how tough it is to get rid of it, I try not to put on five to six pounds above my ideal weight. I weigh myself every morning and if I've gained a couple of pounds, I watch what I eat carefully. Disciplined? Sure I am, but in our fast-food, additive-added, food-obsessed society, no one ever said staying slim was easy.

As for 'grazing', well, I think it's revolting. Cows and sheep graze, adults should sit down at the table and eat their meals in a harmonious and relaxed atmosphere. I find the sight of people walking down the street, munching burgers, eating ice cream and quaffing from cans not only an eyesore, but also exceedingly unhealthy. To process food properly our digestive system needs time, with a break between meals, and this is impossible if it constantly has to work on new amounts of food. Here are some examples of diets from other cultures that I hope will shed some light on the deficiencies of our Western eating habits.

THE JAPANESE DIET

For centuries the Japanese ranked number two in the world for longevity after the Hunzas. They had extremely low mortality rates from cancer and heart disease and the women had a five times lesser risk of susceptibility to certain cancers than Westerners. Today the Japanese have the longest life expectancies in the world. Men and women can live to 78 and 83 respectively.

The reason for their longevity is simple: their diet, which is extremely uncomplicated, low in fat, and consists mostly of fish, rice, cereals, soya, vegetables and a little fruit. Sadly, it has since been discovered that when the Japanese move to the States and start eating American-style food, with their huge portions filled with fat and sugar, their weight goes up, as does their susceptibility to cancer, heart disease and hypertension. It's obvious that these diseases are directly related to diet. Fat-filled, additive-added junk food is the villain. I've always believed that if you eat junk, you'll eventually *become* junk.

THE HUNZA DIET

The Hunzas are an isolated tribe who live in the Himalayas and subsist mainly on fruit and nuts. Like the Abkhazians, the Hopi and Navajo Indians, the Eskimos (Inuit) and the Karakorum, the Hunzas do not suffer from cancer.

The Hunzas eat an enormous amount of apricots and an-individual's material wealth is actually measured by the number of fruit trees he owns. They eat fresh apricots in the summer and dried in the winter. The kernels are pressed for oil, which they use for cooking, for fuel and even as a skin preparation.

In addition to apricots, the Hunza diet includes buckwheat, millet, alfalfa, peas, broad (fava) beans, turnips, lettuce, sprouting pulses and various sorts of berries. The traditional Hunza diet contains 200 times more nitrilosides than the average American diet, their food is poison-free and they may live to be over 100.

Perhaps because the Hunzas survive in rugged mountainous conditions, they have a superior level of health, vitality and longevity to Western man. This may also be because they eat very little protein. Americans consume more animal protein (milk, fish, meat and eggs) than any other nation. Consequently they lead the world in degenerative diseases, heart disease, diabetes, arthritis, cancer and osteoporosis. Now I'm not suggesting you go live in the Himalayas and eat apricots, or condemn yourself to a diet of seaweed and rice for the rest of your long life; but just bear in mind that there is a great variety of foods that are rich in nutrition available – and that what we eat determines the life we live.

IS FAT THE ENEMY?

Well, yes and no. The more fat and the more sugar you consume, the more your body will crave it. But it is important to include some fat in your diet – it just has to be the good type. Fats, such as those used in deep-fried foods like fried chicken, fish and fries, have been linked to cancer and heart disease. Bad sources of fat include butter, cream, fatty meats, bacon and margarine and shortening. These contain trans fatty acids, which may double the risk of heart attack and raise the LDL (low-density lipoprotein – substances, a mix of protein and cholesterol) that carry fats around the body and deposit them in the liver, muscles and on the insides of the blood vessels, leading to heart disease and strokes. HDLs (high-density lipoproteins) are the opposite of this. They carry fats to the digestive system where they are removed from the body. The body needs both kinds: it's the ratio that's important. Saturated fats (e.g. red meat, dairy and lard) increase the ratio of LDLs to HDLs. Unsaturated fats (e.g. oily fish, olive oil and nuts) increase the ratio of HDLs to LDLs.

Strangely enough, you also need to look out for the words 'fat-free' on labels. Take 'fat-free mayonnaise', for example. Regular mayonnaise takes one egg yolk and one cup of olive oil, plus some lemon or vinegar and mustard. In other words, it's 98 per cent olive oil (or good fat). If it becomes 'fat-free,' what's replacing that volume of oil? Labels can prove helpful. Replacements are usually gums, sugars or starches so you'd have been better off with half a teaspoon of the real thing than two tablespoons of fake. The same goes for 'fat-free sour cream', and similar 'healthy foods'.

Just as an excess of fat can cause problems, so too can a deficiency. It's entirely possible to become fat deficient. Among the health problems associated with a lack of fatty acids are dry skin, eczema, low energy, impairment of kidney function, slow infection healing, vision and learning problems, depression, even miscarriage. Use of cholesterol-lowering drugs (usually combined with a low-fat diet) is also associated with a higher suicide rate.

Just to prove you don't need to exist on apricots or seaweed alone, there's an amazing variety of fruits and vegetables that are good for you, and I love them all. (Grayshott Hall, England, 2002)

So, is there any good news about fat? Yes, there are such things as good quality fats. Among the best are extra virgin olive oil (I swear by it), unrefined sesame and sunflower oil, unrefined flax seed oil, walnut oil, organic butter and clarified butter (or ghee). Omega 3 fatty acids are found in fresh dark cold-water fish such as salmon and mackerel, as well as flax seed oil, tuna and some shellfish. Omega 6 is found in sesame and sunflower oil, while fresh organic butter can be an excellent source of natural Vitamin A.

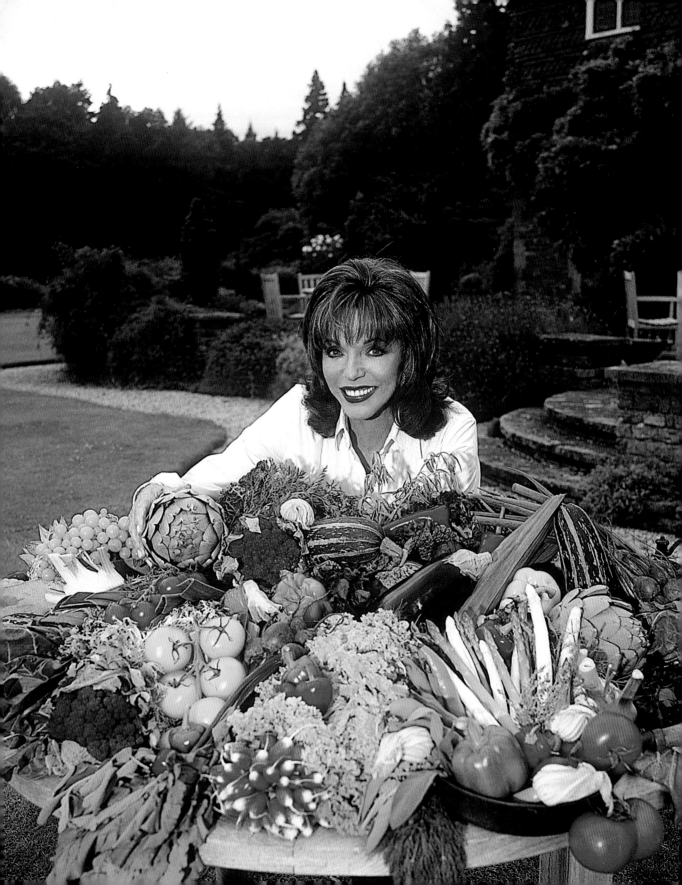

On average, when cooking from scratch about two or three tablespoons of healthy fats, such as olive oil, per day will give us all the essential fatty acids we need. At the same time, it's important to avoid deep-fried foods, hydrogenated fats and fats like lard. Fat-free processed foods and snacks will always encourage you to eat too much, increase sugar cravings but keep hunger unsatisfied. Good-quality fats are beneficial for your skin, hair, nails, immune system, heart, liver and nerves. They also make you feel satisfied when you've eaten.

BAD NEWS FOR FRY-UP FANS

The latest health scare from scientists is that frying, baking, barbecuing and roasting foods creates acrylamide, a chemical which has been shown to cause cancers in laboratory rats and may cause brain problems for humans as well. They go so far as to call it a 'probable human carcinogen'. This is not good news for people who like a fry-up! The British Retail Consortium and the Food and Drink Federation were horrified enough to issue a statement expressing their concern about the possible perils of baking and roasting, 'Manufacturers and retailers are committed to working to establish the significance of these findings for public health and to reduce consumers' exposure.'

LIFE IS SWEETER FOR CHOCOHOLICS

Now for some great news for chocolate lovers. American researchers recently revealed that the treat favoured by millions not only tastes delicious, but it's also good for you. Carl Keen, a nutritionist at the University of California says: 'More and more, we are finding evidence that consumption of chocolate that is rich in flavonoids [70-80% of cocoa solids] can have positive cardiovascular effects.' Flavonoids can help maintain good circulation, a healthy heart and reduce blood clots, a cause of shown that chocolate consumption caused an increase in blood antioxidant capacity within two hours. Antioxidants are believed to help to protect the body from the effects of free radicals that are suspected of contributing to a host of chronic diseases. So, as Carl Keen said, 'Chocolate may contribute to a healthy, well-balanced diet.' As I'm a devout chocoholic, I'm thrilled by the news.

FEEL (AND LOOK) FABULOUS

Here are some more of my personal tips to help you lose weight and feel great.

Go for a walk or run. Exercise can suppress the appetite for at least an hour afterwards. Even a ten-minute walk can stave off the morning munchies and of course it burns calories, too.

Don't waste your money on procedures that are supposed to 'cleanse' the system and promote weight loss. While high volume enemas may be all the rage in Hollywood, there's no evidence that colonic irrigation is helpful and if it's incorrectly done, it can cause an infection, poke a hole in your bowel wall or cause horrible stomach cramps. But there are several ways to detox your system when you've eaten too much or overdone the booze or ciggies (see below).

Push yourself away from the table before you've finished everything on your plate – an excellent exercise!

Have a fast once or twice a year. Confine it to fresh fruit or vegetable juice, which can be diluted in water but don't fast for longer than two or three days. Plan a quiet time at home to do this, avoid alcohol altogether and don't drive while fasting (it affects your concentration levels). This is not suitable for diabetics or pregnant women. If you are suffering from a serious or chronic condition, seek medical advice first.

I've already said don't drink fizzy drinks with your meals. Even seltzer water has bubbles that bloat. A glass of wine is a healthier option and makes dinner (and lunch) taste better. The French swear by it and their saying, 'A day without wine is like a day without sunshine', is certainly true as far as I'm concerned.

Stop snacking. Count up all the bits you've scoffed during the day and you'll be amazed at how the calories mount up.

Try steaming or stir-frying your food. It's much healthier than getting out the deep-fat fryer.

If you feel like a snack, brush your teeth with mint toothpaste or chew a piece of sugar-free gum instead.

Stop eating before you start to feel full.

Keep a food diary for a week and write down what you eat and the calorie content. Remember the recommended daily allowance of calories is 2,000 for women and 2,500 for men.

As a healthier option, I eat a lot of Mediterranean-style food cooked in olive oil with plenty of vegetables and I try to stay away from all fried food, although I enjoy the occasional treat.

I eat red meat, but only twice a week. However, lots of people don't eat it at all, in which case I suggest you take iron supplements.

MY EATING OUT SECRETS

Now, just to show you how much I love to eat, here are a few of my favourite dishes from restaurants I regularly go to. I dine out at least two or three times a week but remember, I only eat a little over one-third or half of what's on my plate. Believe me, it works.

Salmon Fishcakes with Sorrel Sauce SERVES 8

650g (1lb 7oz, 2½ cups) dry mashed potato (no butter or milk added)
650g (1lb 7oz, 2½ cups) salmon fillet, poached in fish stock and flaked
2 tablespoons tomato ketchup (catsup)
2 teaspoons anchovy essence (paste)
3 teaspoons English mustard
salt and freshly ground white pepper
a little plain (all-purpose) flour
oil for frying
1.5kg (3lb 4oz) spinach, picked over, washed and dried

for the sauce
500ml (18fl oz, 2 cups) strong fish stock
50g (2oz, ¼ cup) butter
30g (1oz, ¼ cup) plain (all-purpose) flour
50ml (2fl oz, ¼ cup) dry white wine
250ml (9fl oz, 1 cup) double cream
  (heavy cream)
15g (½oz, ⅓ cup) fresh sorrel, shredded
salt and freshly ground white pepper

To make the fishcakes, mix together the potato, half the poached salmon, the tomato ketchup, anchovy essence, mustard and seasoning until smooth, then fold in the remaining salmon. Mould the mixture into 8 round cakes and refrigerate for 1–2 hours.

To make the sauce, bring the fish stock to the boil in a thick-bottomed pan. In another pan, melt the butter and stir in the flour. Cook very slowly over a low heat for 30 seconds, then gradually whisk in the fish stock. Pour in the white wine and simmer for 30 minutes until the sauce has thickened. Add the cream and reduce the sauce until it is of a thick pouring consistency, then stir in the sorrel and season. Preheat the oven to 200°C (400°F/gas mark 6).

Lightly flour the fishcakes and fry them until they are coloured on both sides, then bake for 10–15 minutes.

Warm a large saucepan over a medium heat. Add the spinach with no extra water, season lightly with salt and pepper and cover tightly with a lid. Cook for 3–4 minutes, stirring occasionally, until the leaves are tender. Drain well in a colander.

To serve, put some spinach on each plate, then a fishcake and pour over the sauce.

(FROM LE CAPRICE RESTAURANT, LONDON)

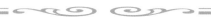

Wolfgang Puck's Classic Chinois Chicken Salad SERVES 4

450g (1lb, 2 cups) chicken breasts (roasted, cooled and
    skin removed), cut into julienne strips
1 head Chinese leaves (napa cabbage),
    cut into julienne strips
2 heads radicchio, cut into julienne strips
225g (8oz, 2 cups) spinach, cut into thin julienne strips
1 head cos (romaine) lettuce, any soft green leaves
    discarded, cut into julienne strips
wonton strips to garnish*
peanut oil for frying

for the vinaigrette
2 bunches spring onions (scallions) (white portion only)
50g (2oz, ⅓ cup) pickled ginger*
25g (1oz, ¼ cup) Chinese mustard powder
120g (4oz, ½ cup) shallots, chopped
80g (3oz, ⅓ cup) honey
150ml (5fl oz, ⅔ cup) good-quality soy sauce
150ml (5fl oz, ⅔ cup) ginger vinegar*
500ml (18fl oz, 2 cups) peanut or vegetable oil
3 tablespoons sesame oil
125ml (4fl oz, ½ cup) chilli oil
salt and freshly ground black pepper

Place the first seven vinaigrette ingredients in a blender, cover and purée for 90 seconds (it may be necessary to do this in two batches if your blender isn't large enough). While the blender is still running, slowly drizzle in the three oils until the vinaigrette is thick and has emulsified completely. Check the seasoning and adjust as necessary.

To make the fried wonton strips, heat the peanut oil to 180°C (350°F) and cut the wonton skins into strips 6mm (¼in) thick. Sprinkle the strips, so that they separate, into the hot oil and fry until crisp and golden. Drain on kitchen paper towels, then lightly salt. Allow to cool before using.

To make the salad, combine the chicken and all the different leaves in a large bowl. Add tablespoons of the vinaigrette, tossing the salad in between additions until well coated but not overdressed. Transfer the remaining vinaigrette to a sealed container and refrigerate for use in other recipes.

Divide the salad between 4 chilled plates and garnish with the fried wonton strips.

(FROM SPAGO RESTAURANT, BEVERLY HILLS)

* Wonton skins, pickled ginger and ginger vinegar are all items that can be obtained from Asian shops or possibly from the Asian section of your supermarket. Pickled ginger and ginger vinegar are usually sold as one product (the ginger is marinated in the vinegar) called 'gari'.

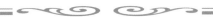

Thai Baked Sea Bass with Fragrant Rice   SERVES 8

You can sometimes order banana leaves from a good Asian or exotic greengrocer.
If that fails, wrap the fish in foil or greaseproof paper (parchment).

for the dipping sauce
5 teaspoons sesame oil
1 small red chilli, seeded and finely
    chopped
2cm (¾in) piece fresh root ginger
    or galangal, peeled and finely chopped
1 stick lemon grass, peeled with the
    bulbous ends finely chopped
3 lime leaves
2 cloves garlic, peeled and crushed
125ml (4½fl oz, ½ cup)
    sweet soy sauce
100ml (3½fl oz, ⅓ cup)
    light soy sauce

for the fragrant rice
2 sticks lemon grass,
    peeled and bulbous
    ends crushed
8 lime leaves
1.5 litres (2¾ pints,
    7 cups) salted water
225g (8oz, 1¼ cups)
    basmati rice, washed
    twice in cold water

for the sea bass
2–3 tablespoons sesame oil
3 medium chillies, seeded and roughly
chopped
2–3 sticks lemon grass, with the bulbous
ends roughly chopped
4cm (1½in) piece fresh root ginger or
galangal, peeled and roughly chopped
4 cloves garlic, peeled and crushed
8 lime leaves, roughly chopped
15g (½oz, ⅓ cup) fresh coriander (cilantro)
8 x 200g (7oz) pieces sea bass, scaled and
filleted
1–2m (3–6ft) banana leaf

First, make the dipping sauce. Heat the sesame oil in a pan and fry the chilli, ginger, lemon grass and lime leaves slowly with the garlic for 1 minute to soften and release the flavours. Add both soy sauces, bring the mixture to the boil, then cool and pour it into a bowl or, ideally, individual soy dishes.

To make the fragrant rice, simmer the lemon grass with the lime leaves in the salted water for 10 minutes. Add the rice and simmer for 10–12 minutes until it is just cooked. Drain in a colander, then return to the pan, cover and leave for 10 minutes before serving. This will help the rice become nice and fluffy. Serve in individual bowls or put it in a large bowl to pass round.

While the rice is cooking, prepare the fish. Preheat the oven to 200°C (400°F/gas mark 6). Heat the sesame oil in a pan and fry the chillies, lemon grass, ginger, garlic and lime leaves for a couple of minutes. Then put them into a food processor with the coriander and chop finely. Spread the paste over the sea bass fillets and wrap each one in a piece of banana leaf like a parcel, folding the leaf so that the edges join underneath the fillet. Bake for 10–15 minutes.

Serve the fish on individual plates with the dipping sauce and fragrant rice.

(FROM THE IVY RESTAURANT, LONDON)

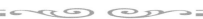

Boulangerie Omelette

SERVES 1

1 small or ½ regular potato, boiled, peeled and cut into cubes
½ small white or ¼ regular onion, thinly sliced and lightly sautéed in butter
2 slices of bacon, fried until crisp and crumbled
3 eggs
1 tablespoon milk or water
1 tablespoon unsalted butter
2 tablespoons grated cheese
salt and freshly ground pepper

The trick to the best omelettes in New York, says the chef of Madame Romaine de Lyon's fabulous restaurant, which serves over 2,000 different kinds of omelette, is to cook the eggs over a high heat and a 20cm (8in) Teflon pan is what he recommends. Make sure you keep the potato, onion and bacon warm on the side until it's time to use it.

Beat the eggs well, then add the milk (or water for a lower fat alternative) for a smoother texture, as well as salt and pepper to taste. Melt the butter in the pan over a high heat but don't allow it to brown. Pour in the egg mixture. Over a very high heat, the eggs should start firming up in about 5 seconds. With a spatula, lightly push the set edges towards the middle to allow the liquid egg to run on to the pan.

When the omelette is almost set, quickly scatter over the potato, onion and bacon and then the cheese. Flip the two opposite sides of the omelette up towards the middle. Slide the omelette out of the pan right on to a hot plate. Simply delicious.

(FROM MADAME ROMAINE DE LYON, NEW YORK)

'21' Cold Senegalese Soup

SERVES 6

Mise en place:
50g (2oz, 4 tablespoons) butter
2 tablespoons olive oil
2 white onions, cut into large dice
2 leeks (white part only), cut into large dice
4 celery stalks, cut into large dice
4 green apples, peeled and cut into large dice
4 tablespoons flour
45g (1½oz, ½ cup) curry powder (Madras brand is best)
1.5l (2¾ pints, 6 cups) white chicken stock
1 kafir lime leaf, finely chopped
1 fresh bay leaf
salt and ground white pepper

Garnish
150g (5oz, 1 cup) cooked chicken breast meat, diced
1 teaspoon curry powder
2 tablespoons chopped celery leaves

Heat the butter and oil in a large saucepan or stockpot over medium heat. Add the onions, leeks and celery. Season with salt and pepper and sauté until translucent (about 10 minutes). Add the apples, stirring to mix with the vegetables, and cook 5 minutes. Sprinkle over the flour and curry powder, and stir until the flour absorbs any liquid. Cook for another 5 minutes, stirring frequently.

Pour in the chicken stock and add the lime and bay leaves. Bring to the boil, then lower the heat and simmer for 15 minutes or until the vegetables are very tender.

Remove from the heat and allow the soup to cool completely. When cold, transfer to a blender in small batches and purée until smooth. Strain through a fine conical sieve (chinois). Taste and adjust the seasoning. Chill well.

To serve, ladle the soup into chilled bowls and garnish with the cold diced chicken. Sprinkle with curry powder and chopped celery leaves.

(FROM '21' RESTAURANT, NEW YORK)

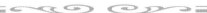

Spaghetti Primavera
Sirio Maccioni's recipe

SERVES 4

1 medium-sized zucchini, cored and cut into 5mm (¼in) dice
½ head broccoli, stalks removed and the florets cut in half
4 fresh porcini mushrooms, cleaned, trimmed and quartered
olive oil
2 garlic cloves, finely chopped
50g (2oz, ⅓ cup) shelled fresh peas
4 green asparagus tips
450g (1lb, 3½ cups) pine nuts, toasted
300ml (½ pint, 1¼ cups) double (heavy) cream
450g (1lb) spaghetti
4 plum tomatoes, peeled, halved and seeded
8 fresh basil leaves, torn
2 tablespoons grated Parmesan cheese
salt and freshly ground pepper

Blanch the zucchini and broccoli in salted water. Cook the mushrooms in a little olive oil in a sauté pan over a medium heat. Add half the garlic and cook until softened. Add the zucchini and broccoli and cook for a couple of minutes. Then add the peas, asparagus tips and pine nuts. Season with salt and pepper and set aside.

Put the cream into a medium-sized pan and reduce by half. Season with salt and pepper.

Cook the spaghetti in abundant salted, boiling water for about 9 minutes. Drain in a colander and return to the pan. Add the cream, then the vegetable mixture, and cook for a couple of minutes or until the paste is *al dente*.

Cook the remaining garlic in a little olive oil in a small sauté pan. Add the tomatoes and cook for less than 1 minute. Remove from the heat and add the basil. Season with salt and pepper. Divide the spaghetti among the serving plates. Top each portion with the tomatoes and basil, and sprinkle with the Parmesan cheese.

(FROM *LE CIRQUE*, NEW YORK)

Plum Tomato and Basil Galette
SERVES 8

This is one of The Ivy's top three most popular appetisers. It is also one of their most plagiarised recipes. It is deceptively simple to make and always tastes wonderful, but be warned, it never quite turns out as it does in the restaurant.

8 x 16cm (6in) rounds of puff pastry, about 3mm (⅛in) thick
240g (8½oz, 1 cup) sun-dried tomatoes in oil
2 teaspoons tomato purée (paste)
8 large or 12 medium ripe plum or well-flavoured tomatoes, blanched, peeled and sliced
freshly ground black pepper
flaky rock or sea salt

for the basil dressing
120g (4oz, 2 cups) fresh basil leaves
150ml (5fl oz, ⅔ cup) extra virgin olive oil

Preheat the oven to 160°C (225°F/gas mark 3). Prick the pastry bases with a fork and bake for 5 minutes, turning them over after 2 minutes to ensure that the pastry does not rise (if it does, you will get an uneven base). Remove from the oven and increase the temperature to 200°C (400°F/gas mark 6).

Drain most of the oil from the sun-dried tomatoes, then process them with the tomato purée in a blender until a fine paste is achieved. Spoon this into a bowl.

To assemble the galettes, spread a thin layer of the sun-dried tomato purée mixture on the pastry bases. Lay the tomatoes in a circle on top, overlapping the slices slightly. Season with freshly ground black pepper and bake for 8–10 minutes.

Meanwhile, wash the blender and then make the dressing. Process the basil leaves with the olive oil, adding a little more oil if the consistency is too thick.

Serve on a warm plate, with the basil dressing drizzled generously over the tomatoes and a pinch of rock salt sprinkled on top.

(FROM THE IVY RESTAURANT, LONDON)

Paupiettes of Black Sea Bass 'Le Cirque'

SERVES 4

Sottha Khunn's recipe

2 leeks (white part only), cut thinly into half-moon discs
100g (4oz, ½ cup) clarified butter
2 large russet potatoes (preferably Idaho) or baking potatoes, peeled and trimmed into 24 large, thick oval shapes
1 x 1.75kg (4lb) black sea bass, cut into 4 x 200g (7oz) rectangular skinless fillets
8 fresh chive stalks

Sauce
10 shallots, thinly sliced
5 sprigs of fresh thyme
225g (8oz, 1 cup) unsalted butter, cut into small pieces
1 bottle Barolo red wine
2 tablespoons double (heavy) cream
salt and freshly ground pepper

To make the sauce, sweat the shallots with the thyme in 1 tablespoon of the butter in a shallow, straight-sided pan (rondeau). Add the red wine and reduce until it has evaporated. Add the cream and reduce again. Whisk in the remaining butter and season with salt and pepper. Strain through a fine conical sieve (chinois) and set aside. Reheat before serving.

Cook the leeks in a little of the clarified butter until tender (about 8–10 minutes). Season with salt and pepper and set aside. Reheat before serving.

Thinly slice the potato pieces lengthways on a mandoline. Toss in clarified butter to prevent them from turning brown. Season the sea bass fillets with salt and pepper.

To assemble each paupiette, lay one slice of potato lengthways on a piece of baking parchment. Place another slice lengthways next to it with a 2.5cm (1in) overlap. Arrange another pair of potato slices over the first two, overlapping half their length. Repeat two more times, to make an oblong shape of eight overlapped slices of potato.

Place a fish fillet in the centre of the potato oblong, making sure that the potato and fish are lined up evenly top and bottom. Starting at the bottom, bring the outer edges of the potato slices from both sides over the fish, one at a time, until the fish is completely wrapped in potato. Brush all over with melted clarified butter and refrigerate for 10 minutes.

Cook the paupiettes in clarified butter in a hot sauté pan, turning to brown on all sides (about 6 minutes in total).

To serve, spoon the leeks on to the centre of each plate. Ladle the sauce around the leeks, place a paupiette on top and garnish with 2 chive stalks.

(*FROM LE CIRQUE, NEW YORK*)

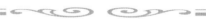

Le Cirque's Crème Brûlée

SERVES 9

225g (8oz, 1¼ cups) packed brown sugar
1 vanilla pod (bean)
900ml (1½ pints, 4 cups) double (heavy) cream

175g (6oz, ¾ cup) caster (superfine) sugar
7 egg yolks

Spread the brown sugar on a large plate or baking sheet and leave, uncovered, until it feels dry and sandy (about 3 hours). Set aside.

Preheat the oven to 150°C (300°F, gas mark 2).

Split the vanilla pod in half lengthways and scrape out the seeds. Combine the vanilla seeds and pod with the cream and caster sugar in a small pan over a medium heat. Heat, stirring occasionally, until bubbles start to form around the edge of the pan. Do not let the cream boil. Remove from the heat.

Whisk the egg yolks in a large mixing bowl. Continue to whisk while slowly pouring the hot cream mixture into the egg yolks. Whisk until the mixture is homogeneous in colour. Pour the custard mixture through a fine-mesh sieve to remove the pieces of vanilla pod and any bits of cooked egg yolk. If you strain the custard into a large measure with a spout or into a jug, the next step will be easier.

Arrange nine 150g (5oz) moulds in a roasting pan with 2.5cm (1in) high sides. Half fill the moulds with the custard and put the pan in the oven. (It is easier to transfer the roasting pan with the moulds only half-full.) Finish filling the moulds to the top; this is important as the custard will lose volume as it bakes. Pour enough hot water into the roasting pan to reach halfway up the sides of the moulds. Bake until the custard is set (about 40 minutes). The custard should tremble slightly when a mould is shaken gently.

Remove the moulds from the pan of water and set on a rack to cool for 30 minutes. Then refrigerate for 2 hours (or up to 3 days). The custards will finish setting in the refrigerator.

Preheat the grill (broiler). Press the dried brown sugar through a sieve to remove any lumps. Immediately before serving, spread a thin even layer of brown sugar over the top of each custard, using about 2 tablespoons for each mould. Set the moulds on a baking sheet and place about 10cm (4in) below the heating element of the grill. Grill (broil) until the sugar is caramelised and light brown. Place each mould on a dessert plate and serve immediately.

(FROM LE CIRQUE, NEW YORK)

Use it or Lose it!

*T*here is no question in my mind at all that next to healthy eating, regular exercise is *essential* to slow down the ageing process. This has been proven by the many people over 50, 60, 70 and 80 who have exercised all their lives and therefore still have the stamina and vitality of their youth. At 80-something photographer Helmut Newton still works for the top fashion magazines and has the zest for life of a man half his age. Actors Gregory Peck and Richard Widmark and actresses Ann Miller and Esther Williams, all in their late seventies and eighties, are incredibly fit and vital. So too are many of my non-actress friends, particularly in the States, who care not to reveal their ages but have the looks, figures, attitudes and vitality of people twenty years younger (and I'm not going to give their ages because I want them to remain my friends!).

Exercise is *the* key and if you don't exercise from the time you are reasonably young you are doing your body and yourself a major disservice. If you are now between 20 and 40, project yourself twenty years into the future. How do you see yourself? As a vibrant, healthy and supple woman who belies her years, or a bent, arthritic and vulnerable old lady who can't get around too well? I've seen women in their late forties and fifties who look like this and too often it's the result of non-exercise. A regime will give you far more of a chance to look like the former rather than the latter. So start now!

I do have Tonia Czerniawskyi, my trainer (whom I affectionately call 'the tiny torturer) who comes to me twice a week when I'm in London but the rest of the time I exercise alone. I'm not keen on going to the gym because it's intensely time-consuming in terms of travel and changing clothes, etc. I exercise on my bedroom floor between 25 and 45 minutes several times a week and these exercises can be done anywhere. I'm not even saying that I particularly *like* exercising. Doing 100 or more sit ups each day can be a crashing bore but I *have* to do them because my body is so used to doing a lot of them that it needs it. But I believe the end justifies the means and I *know* I look and feel good (modest too!).

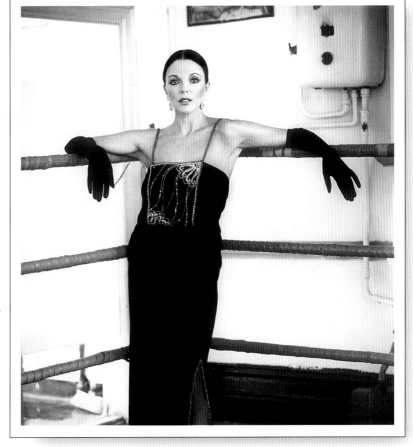

Exercise, moi? Surely you jest? (London, 1980).

THE BENEFITS OF REGULAR EXERCISE

There are many reasons why I exercise on a daily basis:

Exercise combats bone, joint and muscle deterioration and brittle bones are one of the greatest health concerns for older women.

It helps fight bad cholesterol in the same way as eating fibre does.

It burns calories and continues to do so for several hours after you stop. On the days when you don't exercise try climbing (or running) up the stairs quickly.

Exercise gives you a healthier sex life (now *there's* an incentive). Because you feel better, therefore you look better and if you look good, you're more confident about your body.

If you exercise regularly every part of your physique will look better. Your hair will shine, as will your eyes, and your skin has a glow because of sweating which releases toxins and promotes better circulation.

When you begin an exercise regime you become more conscious of your body and therefore you tend to eat better because you're more careful of what you put into it. You just start craving healthier foods.

Regular exercise helps prevent heart disease, strokes and cardiovascular disease, some of the biggest killers of people over 50.

Exercise can stop you shrinking. I have some friends who used to be taller than me, but who are now shorter (and none too happy about it either!).

Exercise helps you sleep. You won't get those insomniac nights because all your muscles will be tired and relaxed from working out.

It makes you happier because exercise releases endorphins into the part of the brain that promotes wellbeing in its pleasure centre.

And lastly, it really does reduce stress and anxiety.

MY FAVOURITE EXERCISES

Here are some of my personal exercises. They are suitable for all ages because they don't put too much strain on the muscles and joints. I've illustrated them with photos of me with my daughter Katy Kass who's in her twenties and does these regularly as well. If you combine these exercises with healthful eating you should see an improvement within a month or six weeks. But exercise alone won't do it. You *must* cut down on what you eat, too.

Wear comfortable clothes and trainers (sneakers) if you want but I prefer bare feet. If in doubt, check with your doctor or physio before you begin and if you feel *any* kind of twinge when doing *any* of the exercises, stop immediately!

Warm ups
These should be done with legs and feet slightly apart. To avoid injury, it's essential to warm up your body before you commence the main exercises.

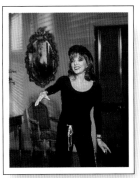 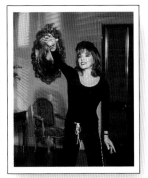 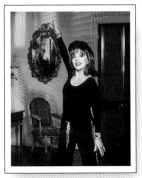 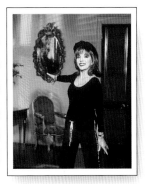

Shoulders/neck
Let your arms hang down loosely by your sides. Start by slowly circling one arm backwards eight times and forwards for eight, then change shoulders. This will loosen up the shoulder joints.

Hold your shoulders up to your ears and then gently release. Do this eight times.

Gently circle your head around, eight times to the left and then change direction with circles to the right.

Trying to keep your balance after a glass of wine is the main benefit of this exercise.

Triceps stretch

An excellent stretch for the back of the upper arm. Start by placing your left hand down the centre of your back as if you were about to scratch it. Now take your right hand and place it on the left elbow. Pull back gently, really stretching, for a count of ten, then change arms.

Chest/biceps stretch

Opposite: Mother and daughter warming up for Swan Lake.

Below: The author applying a Half-Nelson on herself in order to stretch her triceps!

Hold each position for ten counts, stretching slightly as you hold. This is an excellent stretch for the sides of your body.

Lock your hands together behind your back, straighten your arms, tilt your body over and take your hands over as far as they will go. Relax your neck and your shoulders and bend your knees slightly.

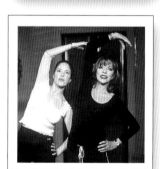

Slowly rolling back up, spread your feet quite far apart and bend over to the right, lifting your left arm above your head and keeping your knees bent. Holding that position, with torso facing front, reach your other arm up and over. Bring the other hand up to meet it and push away. Repeat for the other side.

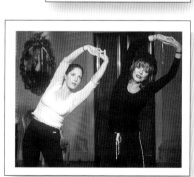

Loosening out your hips and back

Circle your hips round, eight times one way and then eight the other. You should be getting (as opposed to *being*) loose now!

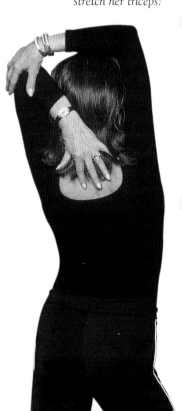

Gentle knee bends

Place your legs widely apart, keep your back straight, place your hands on upper thighs and make sure your knees are in line with your feet. Now bend your knees as far as you can. Repeat at least ten times.

Calf stretch

Facing to the side, one foot in front of the other, lunge forward, bending the front knee. Straighten the back leg and turn the back foot in as much as it will go, so it's parallel with your front foot. Keep your heel down and try not to fall over! Hold for six seconds and change sides.

Quadricep stretch

Holding onto something that doesn't move (a wall, perhaps), grab your ankle and pull it gently up behind you as far as it will go. You will feel stretching in the front of your leg, particularly your upper thigh. Hold for six seconds, then change legs.

Heel raises (or hell raisers!)

This will strengthen the ankles.

Again, holding onto something that doesn't move, lift yourself onto the balls of your feet and then lower yourself back onto your heels. Do this twenty times.

One last stretch (lower back and hamstrings stretch)

If you have a bad back, *don't* do this!

Place your feet together and slowly bend over, pulling in your abdominals. Try to get your arms and hands onto the floor, or at least your fingers to your toes. You can cheat slightly by bending your knees but it's best not to. If you're very flexible you will get down there, but if you're not, you might be lucky to reach your toes!

And that's the end of the warm ups. I must stress once again that it's essential to warm up and stretch before exercising.

Arm exercises

It's very important to tone the arms as they are almost the first part of you to show the signs of ageing.

Biceps

To work the front of the arms, grab hold of some dumbbells/free weights (I like to use five-pound weights). If you don't have your own weights you can use plastic bottles filled with water. Bending at the elbow, slowly raise the weights up and then lower them down. Concentrate on posture, keep your abdominals in and try to think of squeezing those biceps every time you lift the weights up. Work up gradually with more sets as you become stronger. Start out with three sets of five or six repetitions and then work up to three sets of twenty. If you find that you've done as many as you possibly can do with the weights, place them down *carefully* (don't drop them on your toes) and repeat the exercise without the weights for another ten, really squeezing your bicep muscles. Then hold the last one and squeeze even more. Stretch out by shaking your arms, then staying upright, cross your hands together behind your back, straighten your arms and s.t.r.e.t.c.h!

Mother and daughter in a race to the finish.

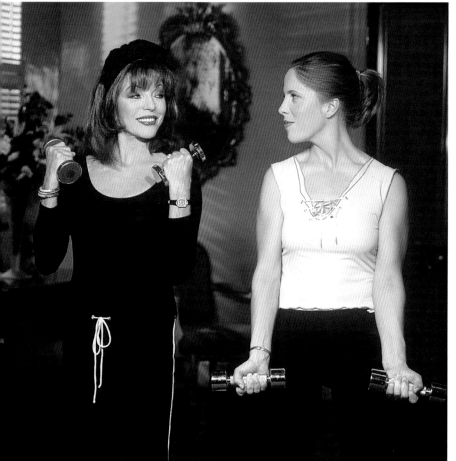

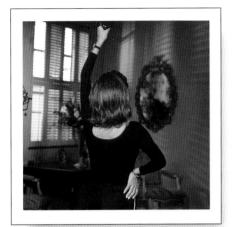 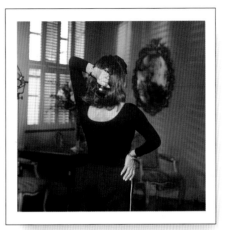

Just trying not to knock yourself over the head with the weight should be strain enough.

Triceps

To work the back of the arms, take a weight with one hand and lift it up and over your shoulder, so that your arm is in much the same position as when you did the Triceps Stretch (only now you have a five-pound weight resting on the top of your back!). Straighten your arm from the elbow, taking the weight up to the ceiling. Do this as many times as you can. Once again you'll have to gradually work up to more repetitions, but try at least one set of ten for starters. Now change arms and repeat. Place the weight down gently and then stretch out using the Triceps Stretch.

This is a great exercise for toning the back of your arms. It's always good to stretch out between sets and after doing each part of the exercise.

'Katy, can you feel your leg…?'

Waist toning and stomach exercises

Repeat Step 3 of the Chest/Biceps Stretch section, but make sure your body doesn't start to droop forward. Keep those abdominal muscles pulled in and reach down as far as you can. Then repeat to the other side. Try and work up to doing 100 of these.

Now you can lie down! The next exercise is very good for loosening out your back. This is definitely one where you might want

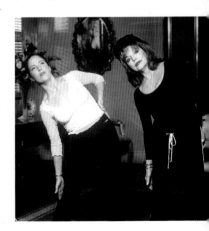

Keeping your knees together, use your abdominals to pull them across your body from one side to the other. I don't usually take things lying down, but I will for this.

to check with your doctor or physio before trying it. If you feel any twinges when doing this – or indeed, during any of the exercises – stop *immediately*!

Knee swings

With your feet together, lift your knees up towards your chest. Then slowly swing your knees all the way over to one side. Then bring them back up to your chest and over to the other side.

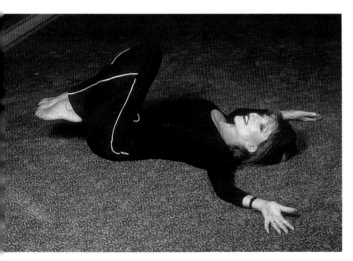
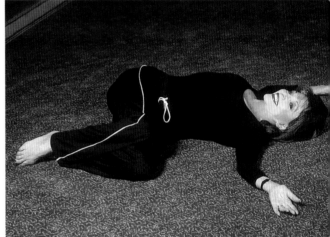

Abdominals

Sit ups

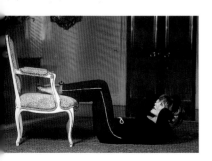

Place your feet up on a chair, knees bent at 90 degrees and tuck your hands behind your head to support your neck. Lift your head and shoulders up as far as you can without straining your back. As you come up, breathe out, and as you roll back down, breathe in. Make sure you pull in those abs every time. Aim to do ten repetitions and on the last one, hold it for a count of three, then gently lower. Take a five-second rest if you need it and then do a second set of ten.

Make sure you don't allow your abdominal muscles to 'pop out'. Pull them in. Almost glue your lower back to the floor! Also, make sure you're not pulling on your neck as you bring your head up. Cycling is a more advanced exercise for the abs. It's basically like pedalling a bicycle while lying on your back, but a bit more strenuous. Remember that all the time you want to pull in the abdominals. Again, place your hands behind your head to support your neck and lift the top half of your body up. Now bring your right knee up while crossing your left elbow over to try and touch it. Then reverse so that the left knee comes up and your right elbow moves across to touch it. Keep your lower back pressed into the floor. Start off with ten and if that's too easy go on to twenty. Try to keep your legs off the floor during the exercise but make sure you are not straining your back. After this you should do some floor stretching.

Do not do this exercise if you have a bad back. You must pull your abdominals in throughout to protect your back.

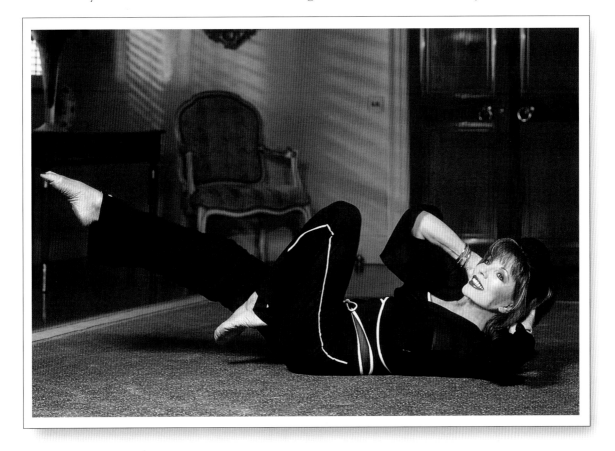

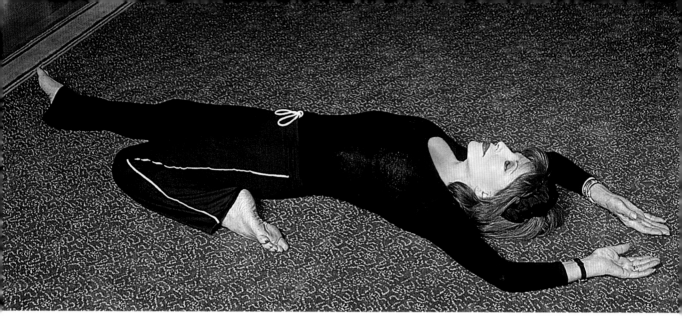

Floor stretches

This is my favourite stretch – which I call the Starfish Stretch. It's excellent for the front of the thighs, but if you have a knee or back problem, be careful with this one and maybe do one of the alternative exercises we did earlier.

Sit down on the floor with one leg back and out at a 45-degree angle, as if you're almost sitting down on your heel. The other leg should be pointing straight out from your body. Slowly lie back (and this is where you could feel a strain on your back, so be careful and use your arms and elbows at first to support you) until your back and neck touch the floor. You can stretch your arms outward at right angles for a bit of a chest stretch. If you're very flexible, you'll look like a star! Now change legs and repeat.

This stretch benefits the back of your legs. Sit up, keeping your legs together stretched out in front of you, and flex your feet. Reach your arms out as far as they go (try and grab your feet if you can) and then slowly bend over as far as you can, using your arms to pull you, until you feel the stretch on your back and the back of your legs.

For the inside of the thigh, stretch both legs out to make as wide a 'V' as you can and then gently bend over in front of you. Don't force anything but hang down as far as you can and you should get closer and closer to the floor. This is a tremendous stretch for the inner thigh.

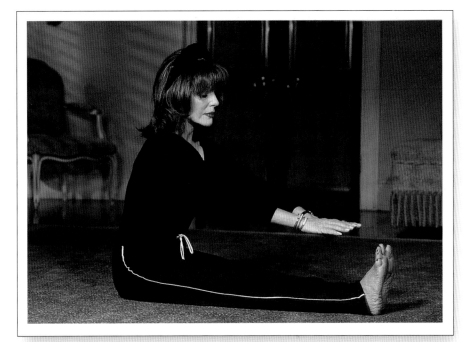

Touching your toes ain't as easy as it looks. If you can't get close to your feet, place a towel around the soles of your feet, grab both ends and gently pull towards you.

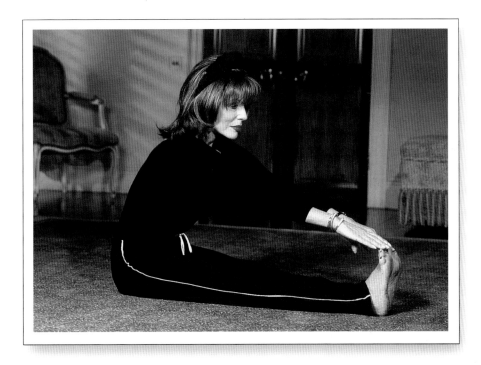

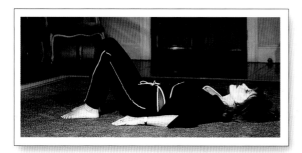 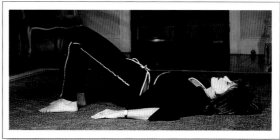

Butt toning exercises

Lie down on the floor and bend your knees, keeping your feet and back flat against the floor. Squeezing your buttocks, push yourself up and lift your bottom three or four inches off the floor. Squeeze hard and gently lower. If you can, try not to quite touch the floor as you go down again. You need to be able to do 30 to 40 of these for them to have any benefit. When you're on the last one, hold it for three counts, keep squeezing then gently rest. If you have a bad back, be extremely careful with this one and only lift yourself up a couple of inches.

For the next stretch, cross your right ankle over your left knee and wrap your hands around your left leg. Keeping your right knee turned out, pull in and you should feel a stretch in your right buttock. Now change over legs and repeat.

*Below: My daughter
Katy Kass, all tied
up in knots… Try to
keep your back on the
floor and remember to
hold the stretch for at
least ten seconds….
And magically
unravel! Don't worry
if you can't get down
this far. It takes time
and practice.*

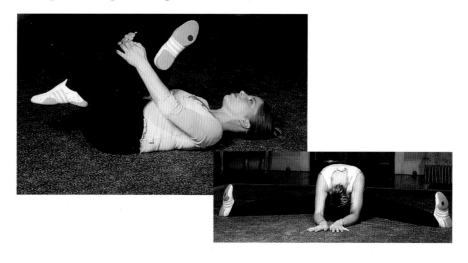

Come up onto all fours and gently swing your right leg in towards your chest, then 'brush' it back out again, trying to swing your leg up above your body as it fully extends behind you. Then pull the leg back in. This should be all one fluid movement. Again, if you've a back problem, be careful with this one and don't swing your leg too high. Start off with ten, then you might work up to twenty. If you're swinging up with your right leg you should feel the tension in your right buttock. Change sides and repeat. Think about your posture (flat back) and holding in your abdominals throughout the exercise. As with all exercise, unless your body is in the right position you won't get the correct benefits, so start by watching yourself in a full-length mirror.

Buttock toning and hamstring exercise. Looks easy, doesn't it? Not!

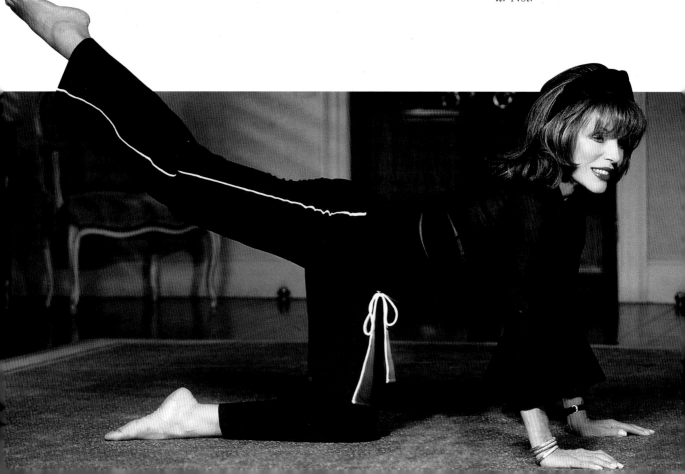

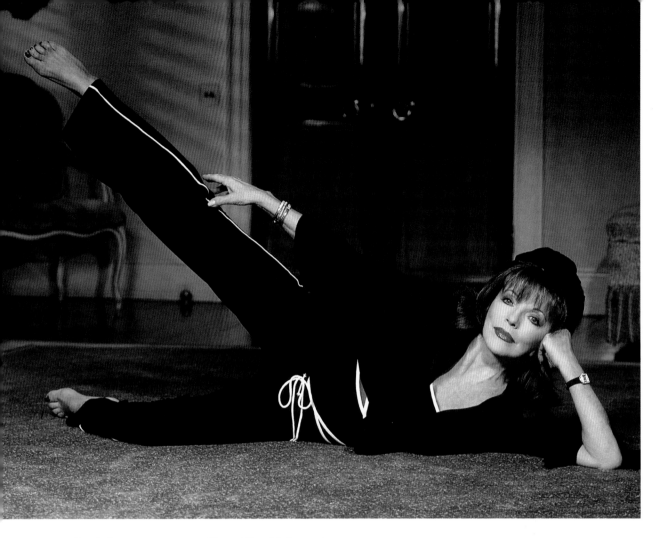

*Don't forget to
control the leg
movement on the way
down as well as on the
way up. (I always
listen to music or
watch television while
I'm working out.)*

Outside thigh toning

Lying on your side, bend your bottom knee and straighten out the top
leg. Lift that top leg up as far as it will go and bring it back down,
keeping it as straight as you can with your top hip forward so you
don't start to roll back. Hopefully, this will also stop the top leg from
coming up high, thereby really working the outside thigh muscle. Do
20 or 30 of these before you change sides.

If you find this exercise easy you might attempt what Tonia
calls 'Little Ones'. Still on one side and keeping your hips forward,
hold your leg up as high as it will go. Now lower your leg down a
couple of inches and just do little lifts in mid-air. If you're doing it
correctly, you will feel that pull in the muscles quite a lot more. Then
finish off with the bigger lifts again.

Inside thigh toning

Stay where you are on your side. Bend your top leg, putting your knee on the floor in front of you, and straighten out the bottom leg. Lift that leg up as far as it will go. Hold it and slowly bring it back down. Some people like to point their foot, others prefer to flex it – it doesn't matter. Try for twenty. Always work on trying to get your leg as high as it will go. As you get tired you'll find this more and more difficult, but keep trying. Again try 20-30 before you change sides. Hold the last one up there for three counts.

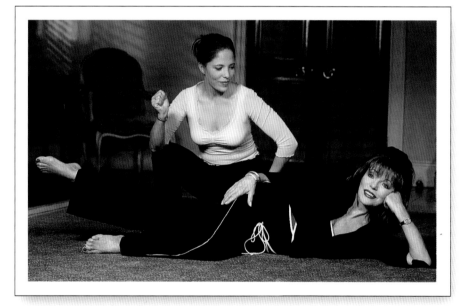

Katy's a hard taskmaster and she works out practically every day. Again, in this exercise as with every exercise, remember to pull in your abs.

When you have finished these exercises (which should take you no more than 20 to 30 minutes), it's essential to do some more stretches. If you have time, repeat the warm-up sequence. If you're busy, just do the floor exercises.

A FEW THOUGHTS ON EXERCISING

I know many people swear by running or jogging, among them my husband, but I am strongly against jogging for women because more and more reports are coming in of the long-term damage it can do. Doctors have reported incidences of muscle fatigue and of joints and cartilages actually wearing out because of too much jogging. It can also cause the breasts to droop and legs to become scrawny. Look at Olympic runners. They all have rather skinny angular legs, not shapely at all. It has also been proven that you can burn off just as many calories when you *walk* a mile as when you run it. Although I know that walking is an excellent exercise, unless I'm window-shopping, I must admit I find it rather boring. What's more, since I live in a city I'm not keen on breathing in even more pollutants, toxins and emissions from vehicles.

One thing I *do* advocate most strongly however is stretching. I stretch first thing in the morning in bed when I wake up, then once I'm out of bed and at various times during the day, particularly when I've been sitting for long periods (like *now!*). By the way, exercise techniques have changed a great deal over the years. It used to be 'no pain, no gain', or 'feel the burn', but not anymore. Regular and reasonably gentle exercise is much more beneficial and there's far less reason to pull a muscle or tendon.

If you're too busy for a full-scale or half-hour work out, just fit in a few bits and pieces throughout the day and it will add up to the full half hour. I myself have grabbed the odd 50 sit ups during a lull on a busy day on set, while in full make-up and costume. I don't suggest you do this every day, but doing *something* is always better than nothing.

One morning, while waiting for a lighting set-up on *Dynasty* and dressed in full regalia – hat, veil and cinch-waisted power suit – I picked up two plastic bottles of water and did a full set of arm work outs to the amusement of the crew. 'It's better than sitting around watching you guys work,' I joked. Another thing I always do is to walk up the stairs. People are amazed that I won't take a lift if my destination is below the fifth floor but that's one of my work outs for the legs and it works!

I can't remember ever not taking exercise. As an infant I regularly went to dancing school, appearing onstage at the age of three and a half. At my schools sports and gym were compulsory. I didn't particularly adore netball or lacrosse but as my mother said, 'It's good for you,' which was one of her favourite sayings as she ladled great tablespoonfuls of cod-liver oil and concentrated orange juice down our gullets. Exercise became a way of life for us and as I entered my mid-teens and became a mini disco diva, I've never stopped. Dancing is a fabulous work out and if you regularly dance the night away, you don't need to do much else.

The only time I ever stopped exercising was when I became pregnant and indulged myself totally in all the foods I craved, like fudge and pecan pie. Consequently, with my first child, Tara, I gained 30 pounds. That was a shock to my system (and my wardrobe) so I started exercising again in earnest and carefully watched my diet (I had also stopped smoking when I was expecting). A year later, pregnant again with my second child, I was back to my fighting weight and believe me, I did *not* gain more than eighteen pounds that time and was back in my old clothes within a month.

Maintenance: skin, hands, nails & hair

As everyone knows, the skin is the largest organ of the body and the one that shows the most signs of wear and tear and age. Consequently it's the part of your body that needs the utmost maintenance. You can always disguise your figure with clothes and your hair with a hat, but it's pretty hard to hide the skin on your face and hands. This is what gets attacked the most from exposure to the elements, particularly the hands.

Being naughty and allowing the Jamaican sun to spread its rays on that pretty twenty-year-old face. I soon stopped when I discovered how destructive it could be.

One often sees a woman who has taken scrupulous care of her face but not bothered with her hands and they show the first signs of age with liver spots, veins and wrinkles. Taking care of the hands is really difficult. In days gone by women wore gloves for maximum protection whenever they went out. Who can do *that* today? You won't die from old skin but it's best not to let it get worn-looking too fast. So let's start with the skin on the face and its major enemies:

The most destructive element your skin faces is the pollution and toxins in our atmosphere. Unless you go to live in the Himalayas with the Hunzas, it's impossible to avoid this. The air that we breathe in, particularly in the city, is filthy and filled with invisible particles caused by emissions from cars, lorries, airplanes, factories and even road works. These invisible enemies attack the skin and inflame it, which leads to the formation of free radicals in the cells. Free radicals attack your body's DNA, the material carrying genetic information, which causes age spots, wrinkles and redness. It is important, therefore, to take antioxidants, which destroy free radicals.

The second enemy is the sun. Keep your face *out* of it and between 11 a.m. and 3 p.m. avoid the sun altogether. Dermatologists estimate that 90 per cent of skin ageing is caused by over-exposure to ultraviolet rays. There's nothing more damaging than those gorgeous golden rays, I know – I love them. I love lying in the sun and so have a certain amount of skin damage to prove it; but since I was twenty, never *ever* have I let those rays touch my face. I wear a sun hat, moisturiser and sun block with UVA (ultraviolet radiation), plus a make-up base and sunglasses.

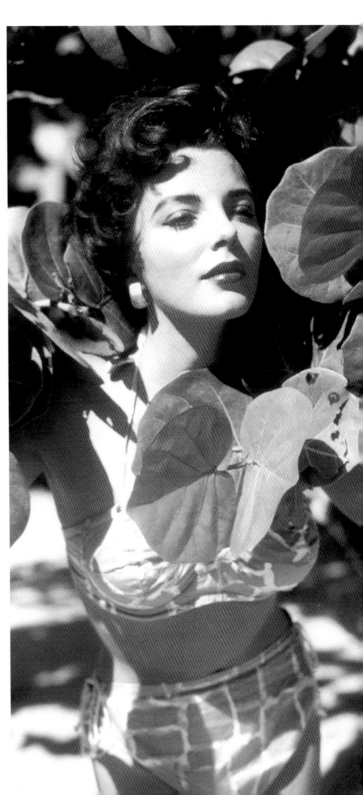

I always think I'm unrecognisable. However, even though I thought there was no one in sight, a paparazzo managed to snap me unawares. Contrary to what many people have said I was *not* posing and was staring into space, considering whether to join Percy on his jet ski. When I finally decided to get on, I promptly fell in, losing my hat, my sunglasses and my poise. Glad the pap didn't get that!

Unfortunately, it's not only the sun that damages the skin these days. The air around us is filled with a terrifying cocktail of toxic substances, all of which are tremendously harmful to your face. Depending on where you live and how industrially built-up your area is, there could be a destructive emission of sulphur dioxide, lead, mercury or zinc poisons, pesticides and carbon monoxide. These are not healthy substances to expose your skin to so if you *really* want to protect your face, cover it up as much as you can.

Smoking: the ultimate killer for the skin, and passive smoking is almost as bad. Each cigarette contains 7,000 or 8,000 free radicals and nicotine makes blood vessels contract so the blood can't get to your skin and nourish it. Smoking also causes horrendous wrinkles around the mouth. Take a look at a friend who's a heavy smoker and you'll see what I mean.

'Oh, but I've seen you with a cigarette,' I hear you say. True, I do smoke, but in extreme moderation, and never more than five or six a day. I usually only smoke in the evening and rarely at home. I try not to inhale or wrinkle up my lips, and I only smoke less than half the cigarette, a habit I picked up from Bette Davis when I worked with her. So basically although I smoke less than three cigarettes a day, I *am* aware of the toxins and their horrible effects, so I'm *trying* to cut my three-a-day habit and when (and *if*!) my husband gives up, I will, too.

I don't pretend to be perfect and the occasional social cigarette gives me pleasure. A doctor told me, 'Smoking less than six cigarettes a day is the equivalent of breathing in the toxic emissions from vehicles if you live in a city.' I'm not in any way condoning smoking –

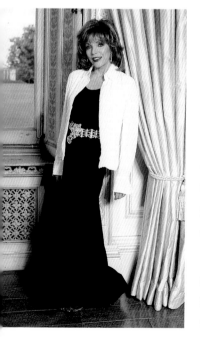

Thrilled at having successfully quit smoking for over two weeks. (Grayshott Hall, 2002)

it's a habit that will lead to certain death. But once again, if you *must*, be disciplined about it. Who knows, you may even end up quitting for good. I always quit smoking when I was pregnant and I *never* smoked around my children when they were small.

Excess alcohol consumption dehydrates your skin and exacerbates skin conditions like psoriasis. If you have a tendency to bruise, alcohol makes it worse, too, and gives you nasty red veins over your cheeks and nose if you imbibe too much over the years. Think what W C Fields looked like after a lifetime of boozing – broken veins, huge blotched nose, bloodshot eyes and none too steady on his feet.

I've worked with some notorious boozers during my career but two stand out in my mind for being able to get totally sloshed while still being able to do a fine job of thesping. Trevor Howard and I were shooting a mediocre epic at Pinewood Studios called *The Bawdy Adventures of Tom Jones*. The bar at Pinewood is a convivial and crowded spot for pre-lunch drinks and Trevor would hold forth there, telling outrageous tales and downing countless 'bevvies' while his enthralled audience of actors and technicians from the movies currently shooting looked on. One day he missed lunch altogether and was so drunk he could barely stand against the bar. When the AD (assistant director) summoned him on set for his scene, I and several other actors watched in some amusement as the old thesp staggered out of the bar.

'He'll never make it,' whispered Nicky Henson, who played Tom. 'He can't even stand up.' 'Let's go see,' I suggested and off we trawled to stand behind the camera and watch the proceedings. I couldn't believe my eyes when Trevor appeared on set, clear-eyed and seemingly sober and performed the scene word perfectly. However, in between takes he collapsed into his chair demanding coffee. It was a *bravura* performance but I think that the excess drinking contributed to the flu and bronchitis that eventually killed him.

I think that was also true of Richard Burton, whom I had

adored since I was a teenager and saw him on stage in *Ring Round the Moon*. I was thrilled to be cast opposite him in *Sea Wife*, which was shot in a glorious location in Jamaica. Close up, Mr Burton wasn't nearly as attractive as he looked on stage. The years of heavy drinking had taken their toll and although he was only in his mid-thirties, his eyes were bloodshot and his skin had a greyish pallor with lots of broken veins. I was amazed at his capacity for liquor. At the end of the day's shooting, when cast and crew would fraternise in various island *boites*, he matched everyone glass for glass and although he got away with it then, eventually his drinking contributed to his early death from a brain haemorrhage at 58.

But one drink that you can never have enough of is water! Drink six to seven glasses of H_2O a day, especially if you suffer from dry skin or eczema. According to Professor Nick Lowe, consultant dermatologist at the Cranley Clinic, London, 'Dry skin or eczema sufferers have a reduced skin protection against water loss and need to drink more to compensate.' Water is good for the complexion because it keeps the skin smooth, supple, elastic and relatively wrinkle-free. The difference between a plum and a prune is the amount of water they contain. When you are dehydrated not only does it show up in your skin you also feel tired and lethargic, have difficulty concentrating and are more prone to headaches, colds, flu and kidney problems.

Among other no's for healthy skin are too much salt, too many food additives, spicy food or hot drinks (if your skin is really sensitive), junk-food (I find it really depressing that it's so readily available), caffeine (unless in moderation) and saturated fat. Many of these things are hard to avoid but you must try if you want good skin. I know it's hard but try to avoid stress, too.

We are bombarded with skin-care products today, many of which advertise anti-ageing properties and cost a fortune. Studies have shown that many of these claims can't be substantiated medically and it can be just as beneficial to your skin to use Nivea or Vaseline, those time-honoured products you can buy for much less. I swear by the following:

Moisturiser: It's essential, but once a day is not enough. When I'm at home without foundation I apply it three or four times a day.

Make-up base: All the women I know who are over 40, and who have used a light base or foundation most of their lives, have much better skin than the ones who have not worn make-up. I watched two separate television programmes recently in which the writers Marcelle d'Argy Smith (ex-editor of *Cosmopolitan*) and Barbara Taylor Bradford were talking. They are approximately the same age (sixties) but the skin on Barbara's face (an advocate of moisturiser and foundation) was all peaches and cream while I'm afraid Marcelle's was definitely not.

'Oh, it's such a bore to put on make-up,' I hear you, dear reader, exclaiming. Well, it's no more of a bore than brushing your teeth or hair and the benefits can be extraordinary. It only takes a few seconds to apply a base. In the theatre make-up is called 'Slap', the reason being that actors just whack it on as fast as they can. If you have mixed the right colour liquid base for your skin, it can take less than a minute to apply. It's worth it, girls – trust me!

A daily course of vitamins. Vitamin C (1,000 mg) is a natural antioxidant, and Vitamin E, sometimes known as the anti-ageing vitamin, is essential to keep skin supple. Beta-carotene, too, helps to protect skin from the sun, and bio-flavonoids, particularly in berries, help produce collagen which keeps the skin firm, allows fluids to permeate it, delivers nutrients, and takes away waste products.

Eat proper food. It's the key to everything we are, really, particularly the skin. Food is the building block to good skin so eschew junk and fast food and try to eat two or three portions from the following each day:
Fresh fruit, particularly cranberries, lemons, limes and oranges (in the 18th century citrus fruits cured the Navy of scurvy). They all contain

masses of Vitamin C, which is necessary for the formation of new collagen and the growth and repair of skin cells. The quickest and easiest way to eat an orange is to slice it into four quarters and suck it (think Marlon Brando in *The Godfather*). This is best done alone as it's not the most attractive of sights. It's boring peeling and dividing oranges into segments so this is how I get that fresh orange.

Mangoes and papaya are also magic for the skin, as are fresh vegetables, olive oil, oily fish, onions and garlic. Avoid hydrogenated vegetable oils found in cakes, cookies, doughnuts, crisps, fries and margarines.

Splashing cold water on your face for a few minutes every morning is stimulating for the complexion and gives a glow, but please put on moisturiser *immediately* afterwards. Exfoliate your facial skin once or twice a month (unless it's particularly sensitive). I shan't go into the benefits of particular products here. Quite frankly they're all pretty much of a muchness, although I have found some of the more expensive products do work better.

Apply night cream every single bedtime after you've cleansed (and toned if you have oily skin). This is where I *do* believe you get what you pay for. For the past four years I've been using a high priced night cream and found not only an improvement in the quality of my skin but that it also seems to prevent those little lines that creep up on you while you are sleeping. The skin rejuvenates itself while you sleep so this is when a good night cream really will do the job.

Get plenty of fresh air and sunlight (but *not* directly on your face). Those of us who live in major cities are lucky enough to have some wonderful parks, so take a walk. Even if it's only a couple of times a week it gets the blood pumping to your face and it is true that country girls usually have better skins than their city cousins, at least until their forties. In my view, country girls have a tendency to eschew beauty products so unfortunately as they scamper up the age ladder their skin starts to deteriorate more quickly.

Avoid yo-yo dieting. Sudden weight loss and gain results in sagging, stretch marks and wrinkling on the neck and face. If you want to lose weight, focus on doing it gradually to allow your skin to shrink and stretch gently.

Cleanse properly. If you wear make-up, you *must* take it all off thoroughly at night. The misconception that make-up causes bad skin was because often women didn't remove it correctly and subsequently got spots, acne and blackheads.

Give yourself a facial once or twice a month. Again, there are thousands on the shelves and they don't have to be expensive. Read the bumf carefully and choose one to suit your skin type.

Try not to frown, wrinkle your nose and lips, or make any facial expression that contorts your face. However, laughter is great and if you have some little laughter lines, so what? It means you're enjoying life.

Don't sleep with your face squashed into a pillow and try to change your sleeping position each night. That is to say, if you always sleep on your left side, switch to your right sometimes and try not to have your head too elevated. If possible, sleep without a pillow.

Stand on your head! Yes, it's really good for your skin as it improves the circulation. I can't do it myself but I know it is also beneficial to lie down with your head lower than your body with your feet elevated.

Vitamin A has been proven to help prevent fine lines and Retin A – now on the market as 'Retinol' for general use – has also been shown to have actual benefits. Retin A is available on prescription only because it can be an irritant to delicate skins. Check with your doctor first.

Try not to use soap on your face. It's extremely drying and can also cause wrinkles.

Plunge into an icy cold bath or shower once or twice a month (unless you have a heart condition). It closes up the pores and invigorates the skin.

Keep the air in the room where you sleep humid. Air conditioning and heating are killers for the skin as they dry it out. If you can't afford a humidifier, keep dishes or saucers of water on the window-sill or on the radiators to moisten the air.

If you can afford it, treat yourself to a professional facial occasionally.

I tried to instill in my two daughters the benefits of skincare from an early age. They certainly listened and they do use special products to care for their skin. However, neither of them is particularly keen on make-up, although I have extolled the benefits, preferring to look *au naturel*.

PREVENTION, *NOT* INSTANT GRATIFICATION

Your skin will show the ravages of time faster than any other part of your body. Wrinkles are the inevitable badge of age, but you can delay and soften their onslaught if you start preventative measures early enough. And the operative word is prevention because I'm sorry to report that there is no cure once those lines have started their dreaded journey down your cheeks. I don't believe in Botox (botulin toxin type A) injections – all the rage in Hollywood now and one of the deadliest poisons there is. Injecting Botox paralyses the facial muscles that make wrinkles but the long-term effects are not yet fully understood.

Anyhow, the thought of injecting Botox into *my* face is anathema to me. Although temporarily effective, the results of eliminating lines on the forehead soon wear off. You have to repeat the process over and over again. Like millions of Americans and Brazilians you could find yourself financially and psychologically hooked. And contrary to popular opinion, face-lifts and plastic surgery won't get rid of wrinkles either.

HANDS AND NAILS

One of the most important aspects of a groomed look is hands and nails. Fact: by the age of 40, women will have only half the amount of fat cells on the backs of their hands as men. How unfair! Also, the female skin is thinner than that of the male and tends to age more rapidly. If your hands are looking a great deal older than your face then you've been neglecting them. Because they're exposed to the elements more than any other body part except the face they will soon show your age. They also receive more wear and tear than anywhere else except the feet. So give your hands some occasional TLC. Prevention being the better part of cure, here are some tips for good-looking hands and nails.

The author, after having just successfully finished a bullfight!

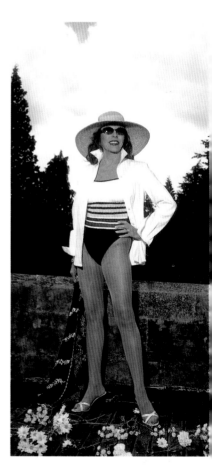

Moisturise after bathing, washing, and after you've done the dishes – in other words whenever your hands have been in soap and water. Keep a bottle of hand lotion next to the sink and rub it in, up to your elbows wherever possible.

Wear rubber or disposable plastic gloves when putting your hands in any kind of detergent for washing up, or for other household tasks like dusting or polishing.

Once or twice a month cover your hands in a rich cream, such as Vitamin E oil or even Vaseline and sleep with cotton gloves on (to save your sheets), and maybe do it when your partner is away! Gloves are available in packets of three at most chemists and drugstores, and are invaluable when you are doing things such as packing and unpacking suitcases, opening parcels or chopping vegetables.

Nails need regular attention. Overdosing on sun or being exposed to very cold air makes them dry or brittle so they, too, need moisturising with a good coat of nail protecting varnish or polish. It needn't be coloured, but polish on nails, like make-up on faces, protects them from the elements and from splitting and breaking.

Doing a DIY manicure? Do *not* use nail clippers as this will make your nails split or break. Also, use a fine emery board instead of a steel file as metal is much too harsh on your nails.

Always push back your cuticles with the help of a good cuticle oil and a Q tip. Never cut your cuticles – they will become ragged.

If you don't like wearing coloured polish, most drug stores sell nail whitening pencils. Apply it under the nails and it looks very effective and clean.

Nails that are too long are extremely hard to maintain and in today's world I think they look a little too artificial. But if you want long nails, there are many nail salons that do brilliant, long-lasting extensions. However, once you've started having silk or acrylic wraps on your nails, you will find you have to keep on doing it as these processes are exceedingly destructive to the nail bed and will start to weaken it.

If your hands are grey and grungy from winter, rub fresh lemon juice over the backs of them and then soak them in warm milk for ten minutes. Try this a couple of times a week until you can see an improvement.

And finally, nothing improves hands and nails as much as a professional manicure. I have several good manicurists in all the major cities I visit and I can really see the difference when I have had a proper manicure and the excellent hot oil treatment that many of the better salons are doing.

We often use our hands to express ourselves so make sure they're saying the right things about you!

SAY GOODBYE TO BAD HAIR DAYS

Hair is supposed to be our crowning glory but unless you take care of it properly, it can start to look like a lank rat's nest. For many women, their hair is the bane of their existence and more money is spent on hair care and hairdressing than on practically any other grooming. Since today's styles are basically 'blow 'n' go' I'm not going to discuss elaborate coiffures here although we are illustrating how styles have changed through the past several decades.

The sad fact is that if you haven't *got* great hair, you're in

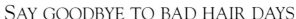

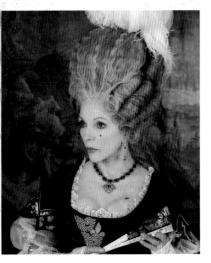

The ultimate bad hair day, this 18th-century fright wig I wore in The Clandestine Marriage *weighed a ton.*

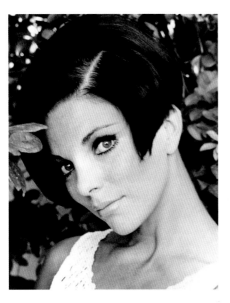
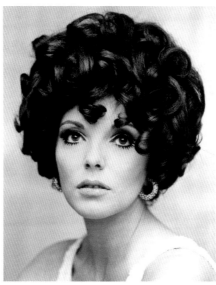
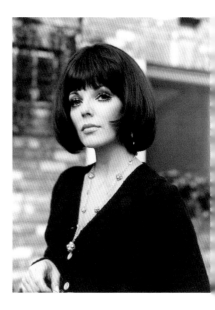

trouble. I'm sorry, but nothing can make thin hair look thick. All you can do is wash and condition with a volumising shampoo. Then spritz with one of the utterly confusing products that used to be called 'Setting Lotion' but now go by various pseudonyms such as 'Revitalising Mist', 'Bounce Back Curl-up Spray', 'Instant Detangler' 'Quick-fix Style Refresher', 'Style Spray & Scrunch' and dozens of others. I go into a complete tail-spin when I'm perusing the shelves of my beauty supply store. There are so many products, it's just the luck of the draw which one will work for you, so keep experimenting and ask your hairdresser's advice, too.

I still believe in good old-fashioned rollers to get a bit of bounce in the hair, but never use hot rollers on fine or delicate hair. They will eventually destroy it, as will a perm. I have found that the less I do to my hair, the better its quality, especially since I stopped the back combing and spraying of the eighties and went for a more natural look. However, I still like to wear hair pieces and wigs sometimes and although they are out of fashion now, my attitude is: 'It suits me, so why not?' The end result is what matters. So my tips

Above left: The sleek Vidal Sassoon bob of the sixties entailed a lot of backcombing and a ton of hairspray, and needed trimming every ten days.

Centre: The soft bouncy curls of the seventies needed big-time setting lotion, and a ton of patience to get this effortless-looking effect.

Above right: A timeless and easy look for thick hair (this is a wig).

...And yes, that's the same mirror from page 18. Entranced by the contour of an eyebrow and always ready to pack (Rome, 1960s).

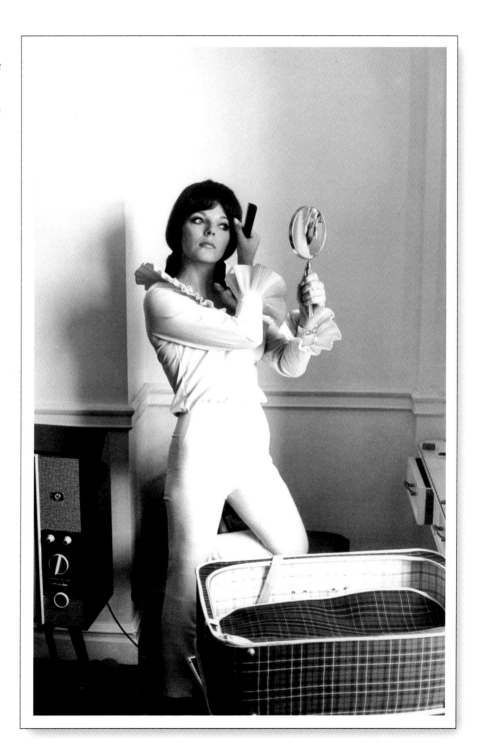

for making the most of your hair are really quite simple:

Shampoo with a non-alkaline product but change your brand every two or three months. Hair becomes used to the same shampoo and doesn't respond well after a while.

I believe 'Head and Shoulders' is the best shampoo to get rid of dandruff. Apply a baby detangler like Johnson's 'No More Tangles' if your hair is thick and curly or tends to get knotted.

Don't condition after every shampoo – it leaves a build-up. I condition every other time I wash my hair.

Try not to blow-dry your hair as this damages it. The best way to dry hair is to let it happen naturally.

Don't use a steel comb or brush. Hair should always be treated gently. The way stylists at fashion shows treat young models' hair – pulling, tugging, back combing and hot-rollering – is shocking. By the time those girls are 35 they could have lost nearly half their hair. On *Dynasty* I insisted on wearing wigs to protect my own hair, not only from the hot lights but also the hair dryers and hair sprays the hairdressers loved to wield. Even the wigs would 'die' every two weeks from the atmosphere and the way they were treated. I noticed the other day on TV one of the actresses I worked with on *Dynasty*, who was lucky enough to have the most lustrous thick hair. The hairdressers *loved* blow-drying it, rolling it up constantly and setting it in elaborate styles. But she was so young, she didn't really care and because of the rough treatments, her hair now looks a great deal thinner than it was.

Have a decent cut but watch your hairdresser while he (or she) is cutting your hair. Hairdressers *love* scissors and not that many of them are real experts in the art of cutting.

And finally, find a style that suits you and your lifestyle, is easy to wear and more importantly, easy to take care of. You don't want to spend hours (or hundreds of pounds or dollars) at the hairdressers so keep it simple, keep it easy and keep it quick.

Making up is not so hard to do

5

Cosmetics have been around since the dawn of womankind and many of our ancestors probably wore more than we do today. Not that today's woman wears much make-up. The current fashion is to look as natural as possible but that is often achieved with a dozen different cosmetic enhancers. It used to be thought that being beautiful was desperately time-consuming, involving hours of painting, primping and preparation. That concept is as old as a Beach Blanket movie. Today's beauty routine should be fast, fun and relatively effortless. Most of all, it must be enjoyable – and using make-up *can* be a lot of fun.

When strolling through the bustling make-up counters in the department stores, I often wonder, who buys this stuff? And where do they put it? In my view, it doesn't look as if many women put any cosmetics on their faces at all. I love cosmetics, always have, ever since I was a little girl and watched my mother applying the foundation, powder and lipstick that not only suited her, but did most women, too.

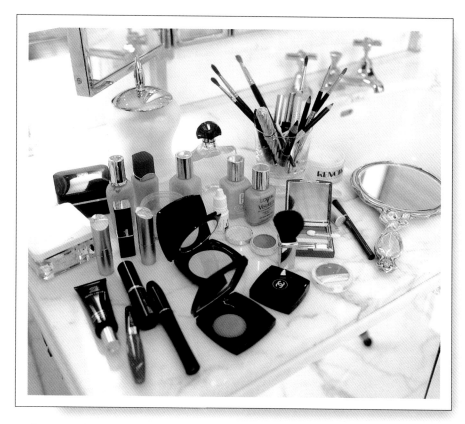

The tools of the trade.

I don't understand why so many women and girls today seem to be scared of using make-up. Do they think they'll look tarty? Do they think it's bad for their skin?

I'm often accused of wearing too much make-up (which in the past I admit I *have* done, particularly in front of the cameras during my *Dynasty* days). However, I can rattle off (but won't!) the names of a number of actresses who wear more make-up than I do. Putting on 'my slap' is my private time. I always have music or the television on, and I often talk on the speakerphone or use the time to think about all the things I'm planning. When I first went to Hollywood shortly after working at Ealing Film Studios in London I was lucky enough to learn how to do my make-up expertly. The difference I saw in the techniques practised in the gleaming hi-tech rooms at Twentieth

Century-Fox compared to the dusty cramped cell at Ealing Studios was enormous. At Ealing I was made up by an ancient old codger called Mr Wilson, who had been making up British film stars since the days of Gracie Fields and George Formby. He only had a couple of foundation colours, which were called No. 5 and 9, two ratty old powder puffs, which were occasionally given a quick wash, and some run-down brushes and eye shadow pencils that looked as though they'd been left over from World War II. His tools were basic and exceedingly unglamorous, his two lipstick colours down to their last dregs, and when he applied my base it was obvious that he hadn't washed his hands. Oh dear! I meekly begged to be allowed to do my own face but he was a martinet and wouldn't dream of allowing such a thing. Since he was in his sixties and I was seventeen, it was a no-win situation for little Joanie.

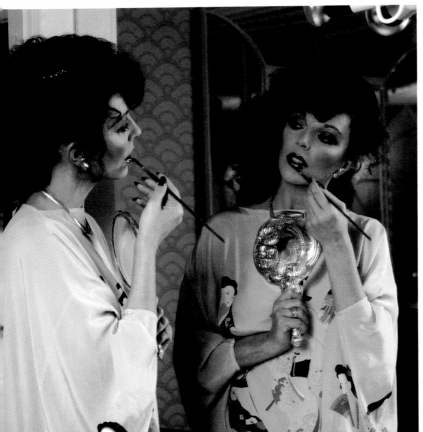

And it's still the same mirror. Author fascinated by the art of lip-lining (London, 1970s).

In contrast Whitey Snyder, the top make-up artist at Fox, was a genius. In his mirrored cave were dozens of jars of foundation in every conceivable colour, twenty different shades of face powder, which he taught me to mix to obtain the correct colour for my skin, shadings galore, hundreds of different coloured eyebrow and eyeliner pencils sharpened to a 'T' and several dozen lipsticks in every colour imaginable. His first job with me was to make my twenty-year-old face look like a seventeen-year-old in *The Girl in the Red Velvet Swing*.

HOLLYWOOD'S BEST-KEPT MAKE-UP SECRETS

I was thrilled when Whitey was assigned to *Rally Round the Flag, Boys*, a movie I was shooting with Paul Newman and Joanne Woodward. One morning he even let me watch him doing Joanne's make-up. Whitey was Marilyn Monroe's favourite, but by now she had gone to the Actors' Studio in New York, so we had him to ourselves for a while. As he painted my face he'd sometimes talk about Marilyn, whom he loved, and we were all fascinated. He told us about a black metal travel case he had designed for her in which to house her extensive collection of cosmetics. It had five drawers and separate sections for foundation, skin, eyes, lips and cheek colours. 'Marilyn knows more about shading her eyes to give herself the "Garbo lid" than I do,' he grinned. ''course, I taught her a lot. When she first came to Fox she wore far too much make-up, particularly her base, which was much too thick and heavy, and she had old-fashioned bright red "bee-sting" lips and unplucked eyebrows. We worked on her look together.'

Marilyn's 'look' was truly original. The shadow above her eyes was as cleverly done as that of Garbo's twenty years earlier, and her face was expertly shaded to give the illusion of high cheekbones. 'Marilyn was beautiful,' said Whitey. 'But when she was in full make-up and hair she was magical. I also taught her to put Vaseline on her face to create the illusion of depth and luminosity. Her eyebrows were plucked and painted into a winged look and we put plenty of shiny gloss over her famous lips, which we made bigger with lipstick.'

Whitey then showed me how to put on my foundation so thinly it was almost translucent and to apply powder thickly but then brush it off to keep it fresh for a twelve-hour day of shooting. Ever since then I have usually insisted on doing my own make-up for films and TV and I know I do it better than the so-called experts would – and faster, too.

'I taught Marilyn how to stick on her Glorene eyelashes,'

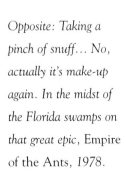

Whitey informed me as he skilfully applied some to my own lids. 'She had a whole box of lashes and they looked like a nest of spiders.' Whitey taught me many tricks, some of which still work today. One of the wisest was: 'Always put on make-up in front of a magnifying mirror in the harshest northern light possible. If you look good in a bad light, you'll look *great* in good light,' said Whitey. Anyway, here are the tips I've learned from the Hollywood make-up experts for applying a perfect make-up (bearing in mind that I'm not into the natural look!).

ON LOCATION

If I'm in a hotel, I never make up in the bathroom as the light is never true. I usually find a nice bright window and lay out my stuff on anything handy – a chair, a desk or a stool. I can put my face on anywhere, and on location I often have to.

It's useful to have two sets of make-up: one to keep in the drawer of your dressing table, the other to have as a travel kit. I try to obtain the little samples of base and blusher that some cosmetic companies give away as an incentive to buy their more expensive products and these are excellent to take to the office or on planes when you travel.

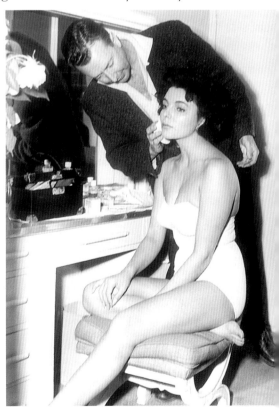

*Opposite: Taking a
pinch of snuff… No,
actually it's make-up
again. In the midst of
the Florida swamps on
that great epic,* Empire
of the Ants, *1978.*

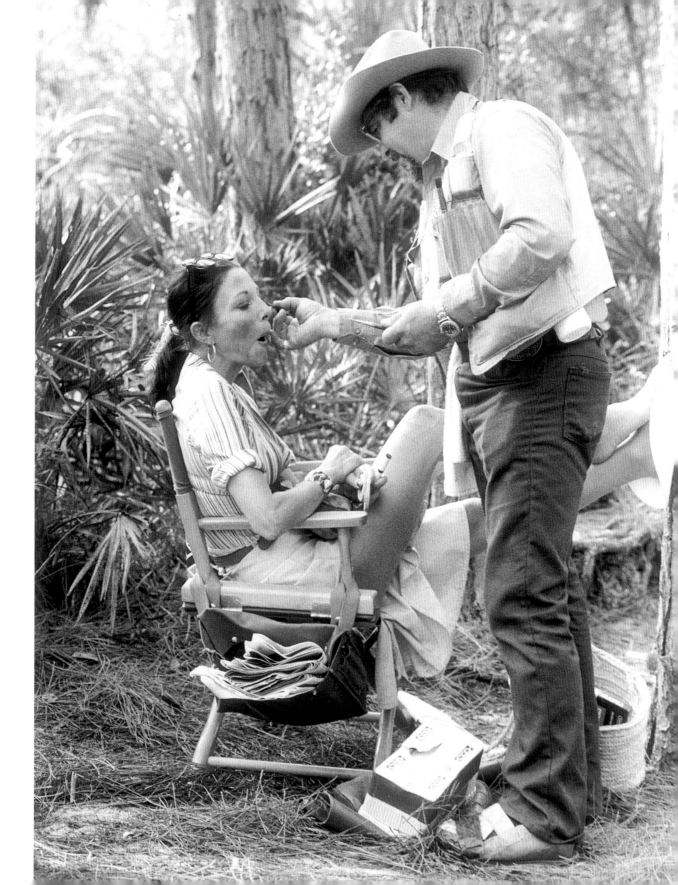

You need a steady hand to apply eye-liner properly. Getting ready to work with Leonard Rossiter for a Cinzano commercial (London, 1982).

I'm not going to tell you what particular brands to buy. To me, they're basically all the same, only the prices, bottles and containers are different. That's why I don't buy too much expensive make-up. Many of the products I use come from the drugstores or professional beauty suppliers in LA and New York, and in London, and are quite reasonable. I *know* that the department store eyebrow pencil can be purchased for far less at a chain store, as can lipstick, eye shadows and base, so why pay those inflated prices?

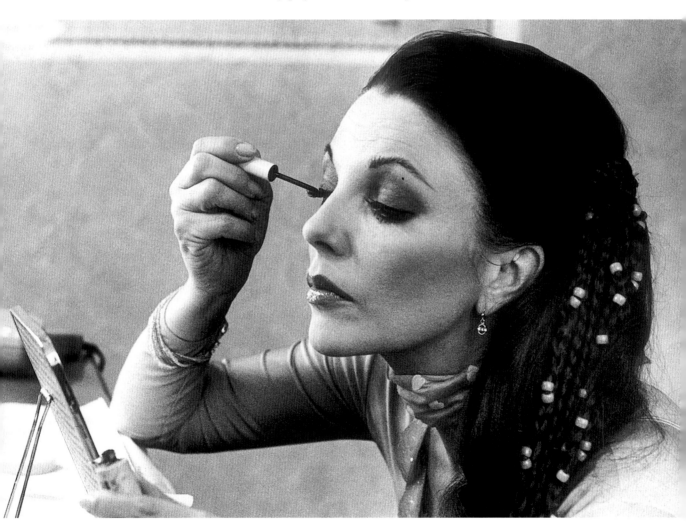

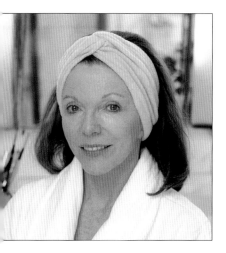 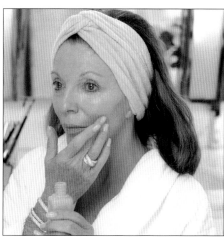 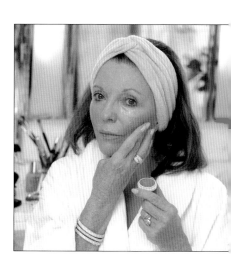

NOW TO THE DETAILS!

First, make sure that your face is clean and non-oily. Use a toner if you have excess oil. I usually apply moisturiser to my cleansed and toned face, then leave it to settle for a few minutes.

Apply the lightest-in-texture liquid foundation and try to get the colour as close to your own skin as possible. I usually achieve this by buying a light and slightly darker base, then mixing them together in another bottle until I get exactly the right colour for my skin. I slap it on fast, dotting it all over my face and rubbing it in with my fingers. Sometimes I use a small sponge but that is optional. Either way, this takes less than a minute.

For dark circles under the eyes or areas of discoloration on the skin, I use a cover-up stick, which I apply very lightly, either with my fingers or with a brush.

Once my face has been covered, I blot it with a folded tissue until all the excess moisture from the foundation has been absorbed and then apply cream blusher under my cheekbone and in the hollow of the cheek, which I also blend with my fingertips. It's important to find a pale-ish colour, but unfortunately most of the blushers today are

Above left: Barefaced and ready to roll.

Centre: Putting on the base.

Above right: Pale blusher under the cheekbones goes next.

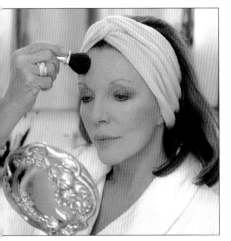 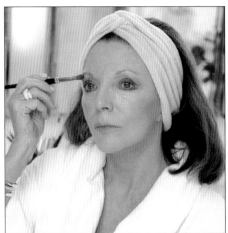 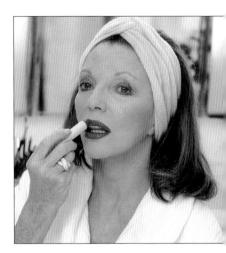

Above left: Keep your powder dry. After powdering, I brush it off with a small brush.

Centre: Powder eyeshadow applied with a sable brush.

Above right: Applying lipsticke.

either too bronzy or too bright pink, so you need to search long and hard. Also, don't ever put anything with glitter on your cheeks, and leave the Popsicle-coloured eye shadows and lipsticks to the teenagers.

I then put a brown shadow pencil around and below my eyes and above my eye socket. The reason I do this is because I have quite a large expanse between my eye socket and my eyebrow, which needs to be shadowed. For this, I use a flat brush. I buy the brushes from a beauty supplier but it is far cheaper to buy sable brushes from an art store and they are usually just as good, if not better.

I then take a small brush and, with the powder I have mixed to suit my skin colour (usually translucent and two shades darker), I powder my face, making sure I don't pull the skin under the eyes. It is essential to blot with a tissue as much foundation from under your eyes as possible because that's what accentuates lines. This is a trick that Whitey taught me and it has served me well. I then remove any excess powder with a small brush.

I'm very fond of bright lips, so I usually outline my mouth with a lip pencil in a colour as close as possible to the lipstick I'm using. (I still contend that lipstick is the most flattering cosmetic a woman can use

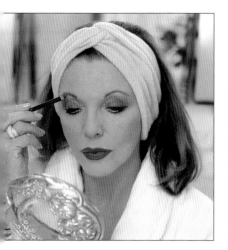 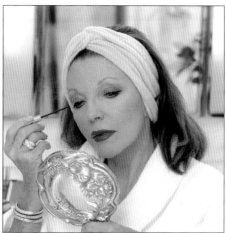 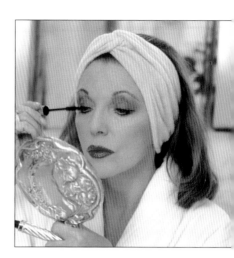

and not only that, it also prevents your lips from becoming dry and cracked.) A big no-no is to have the lip pencil line showing. It's very eighties and I'll admit I was sometimes guilty of it. I fill in the rest of my mouth with lipstick and then, with a lip brush, I go slightly over the top of my upper lip to make it look fuller. I'm not into collagen jabs or silicone plumpers. I think the look of surgically enhanced lips is quite revolting and I feel there are also potential dangers long term. Because my eyebrows were plucked when I was very young (for the movie *Decameron Nights*) and never grew back terribly well, I pencil them in with a medium brown eyebrow pencil and then use a very sharp black pencil to apply tiny lines to simulate hair.

I then play with various coloured powder eye shadows in browns, dark greys, taupes and sometimes black, using a fine sable brush.

Depending on where I'm going, once I've added a quick brush of mascara, this would be all that I would do during the day.

For a more dramatic look to the eyes I use liquid black eyeliner. I've used eyeliner since I was seventeen and I would never give it up. I'm also quite partial to extending the eyes at the outer corners à la Cleopatra, and guess what? The current fashion magazines say eyeliner is back! Hurrah.

Above left: Eyebrows get pencilled in.

Centre: Applying eyeliner.

Above right: Finishing off with mascara.

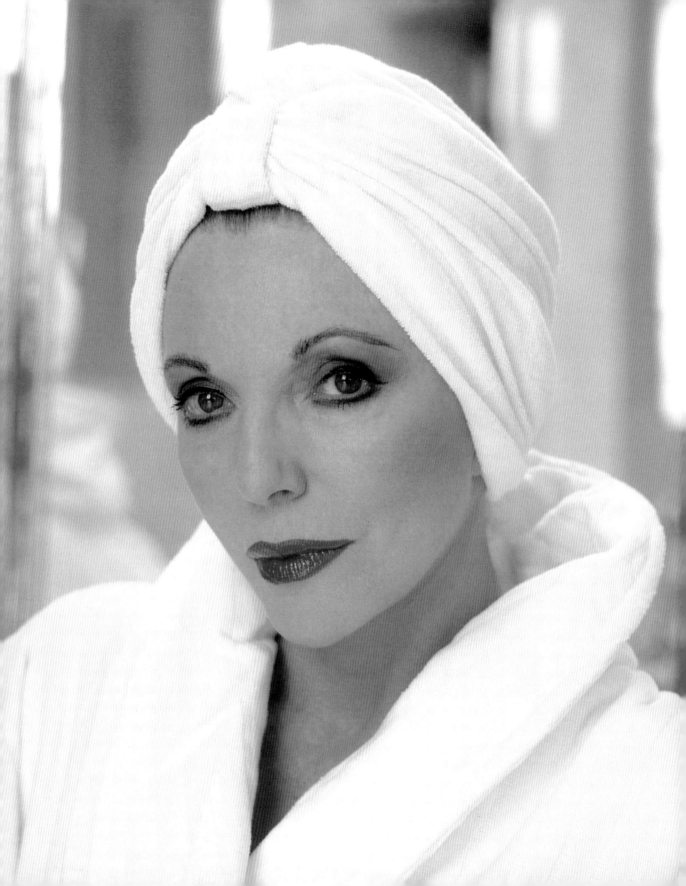

To make sure that your make-up will last, spritz with Evian spray or dab lightly with cotton wool that has been briefly dipped in water.

My finished face, and the whole process took less than eight minutes.

This whole performance takes me anything from four to twenty minutes, depending on how much I daydream. Two last points: one of the essential tools to have is a pencil sharpener so that your pencils are always sharp and make sure that your brushes and powder puffs are always clean.

Once I've applied this make-up I can work in front of the camera for twelve or fourteen hours, and with the exception of re-applying powder, lipstick and eye shadow it will look almost as good at 6 p.m. as it did at six in the morning.

We've all got too much make-up, drawers and drawers full – I know I have. I find it very hard to throw it away and am constantly saying, 'One day I will have a big clear-out.' That day has not yet come, but I'm really looking forward to it. The aim of every woman should be to have your make-up routine down to a quick and fine art. Streamline your make-up drawer and tools and experiment sufficiently to know the good and bad points of your face well enough to accentuate or detract from them as necessary. But remember one thing: make-up can only look as good as the skin that it goes on, so don't expect miracles if your skin is not in good shape.

LIPSTICK PERILS

I love red lipstick and I usually wear it, but it does have its disadvantages. During *Dynasty*, in a scene in which I elegantly blot my lips with a napkin at an exclusive dinner, a huge red stain appeared on the pristine white cloth. The cameraman yelled, 'Cut!' and we had to blot and re-shoot. But they didn't have any more napkins so I had to position it carefully so as not to reveal the blob. I once had a glass of wine at a pub and I left my lipstick imprint on the glass. From then on, the publican displayed it on a shelf above the bar with 'Joan Collins' kiss print' printed on a sign above it!

One disadvantage of female friends wearing lipstick is the endless kissathons we all have to endure at social functions. Recently, an acquaintance gave me a smacker on the cheek and then, showing her excitement at our encounter, dropped her face onto my shoulder to give me a big sincere bear hug. A couple of hours later in the powder room I discovered not only my friend's lip imprint in the middle of my cheek but also a great lipstick smudge on the shoulder of my white suit (which the cleaners couldn't remove). Moral: when wearing lip paint, consider it a lethal weapon sartorially.

MORE THOUGHTS ON MAKE-UP

If you put your make-up on in the morning and have to go on to a party at night straight from work, it's a good trick to remove the make-up below your eyes with cleansing wipes – that's another tip I learned in Hollywood. Quick to use, they give the face a little lift and moisturise it, too. You can then re-apply your base lightly but you won't have to re-apply your eye make-up because you won't have touched them. At the studios they usually do this after ten hours' shooting or at lunchtime.

As far as colours are concerned, I don't think any cosmetics with sparkle in them are flattering and I certainly don't like bright blue or bright green eye shadow on anyone because it looks far too 'barmaidey' and cheap. As I'm a brunette I can use black, grey and brown shading on my eyes but for a blonde or redhead, I suggest substituting brown, auburn and grey. Sometimes, if I'm filming, I use a white pencil just above my lower lashes inside the lid, which makes the eyes look larger and brighter (something all the movie stars of the thirties and forties did).

The whole trick to making up your face so that you look better than nature intended (everyone does – *sorry!*) is not to be afraid to experiment. Most department stores will give you a makeover and a few free samples, and you *don't* have to buy the products. Try it: you'll be amazed at what it does for you and the ideas you can pick up as you go along, and as I've said before, as a foundation afficionado the benefits to the skin in later life are truly remarkable.

Make-up techniques have changed tremendously. When I started out the studios would plaster my teenaged face with thick gloop called 'panstick' or 'pancake'. This was usually of a virulent shade of orange and I hated it. My eyebrows were painted on jet black and half an inch wide, and gooey scarlet lipstick completed the look. Of course this was in the English studios which didn't have the same choice as the American ones. The glamorous female British stars of that era, among them Margaret Lockwood, Patricia Roc and Jean Kent, couldn't match the sheer perfection of the Hollywood actresses including Elizabeth Taylor, Lana Turner and Ava Gardner. Perhaps it was because they didn't have the same vast range of cosmetics, or maybe the American techniques were better. I know after I went to Hollywood eighteen months after starting out in British films I looked a *lot* better. I also looked ten years older than I was. Curiously this was what we all were striving for. Can you imagine a seventeen-year-old today *trying* to look 30? Now it all seems to have been reversed with 30-year-olds wanting to look like teenagers. However, I was encouraged to see pictures of Sharon Stone at a recent Cannes Film Festival. Her classic grooming and elegant wardrobe were nothing less than full-on screen-goddess glamour, something that Hollywood (and the rest of the world) has been missing for far too long.

Glamour & how to achieve it

My *ultimate favourite* glamour queen – gorgeous Ava Gardner.

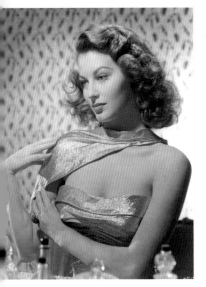

So what exactly *is* glamour? Glamour used to be associated with the occult (yes, really) and denoted an attractiveness that was exciting, fascinating and romantic, almost too powerful to be real. For 30 years, from the twenties to the early fifties, Hollywood gave us true glamour and stars cast a bewitching spell over a world recovering from the Depression and two terrible wars. Today's newspapers and magazines are full of so-called glamour (or 'It' girls as they're known). But to me (and many others) most of these women can't hold a candle to the truly great glamour queens of yesteryear. Ava Gardner, Vivien Leigh, Lana Turner, Jean Harlow, Rita Hayworth, Marlene Dietrich, Greta Garbo, Audrey Hepburn, Marilyn Monroe . . . the list is endless. Each possessed an individualism unique to herself.

These stars genuinely *wanted* to look different from other stars and it would have been anathema to them to appear as a carbon copy of anyone else. Their stylists, costumiers, make-up and hairdressing experts all strove to develop each actress's individual style and woe betide any of them if the actresses were made to look like a 'copy-cat' version of someone else. Of course the 'B' picture actresses copied the big name stars slavishly and each minor movie studio had its own Joan Crawford, Lana Turner or Betty Grable clone but the big stars themselves were utterly unique and inimitable. I am still (more than ever) totally fascinated with watching movies from Hollywood's Golden Age. Every actress looked so stunning and was a complete original. Today, in most British and American movies and soaps, I sometimes find it hard to distinguish between the actresses, who seem to have a sameness or ordinariness about them.

Yes, I *know* it's fashionable today to wear hardly any make-up, to let your hair hang over your eyes and to appear in the most pared-down casual clothes, but I still think that many women look like boring replicas of each other. Even leafing through magazines, I often find it hard to tell the difference between many of the celebrities, who look as if they've been cut from the same cookie cutter.

Fashion magazines seem to want to show their readers glamour (and certainly, many of the models *are* gorgeous) but the pictures in them are mostly unattainable to real women. The poses, too, while exotic and exciting, are unreachable for them. Yet this wasn't the case at all with the great movie stars, who were slavishly admired. Most ordinary women had their favourite, and would often emulate the star's hair, make-up and clothes to suit

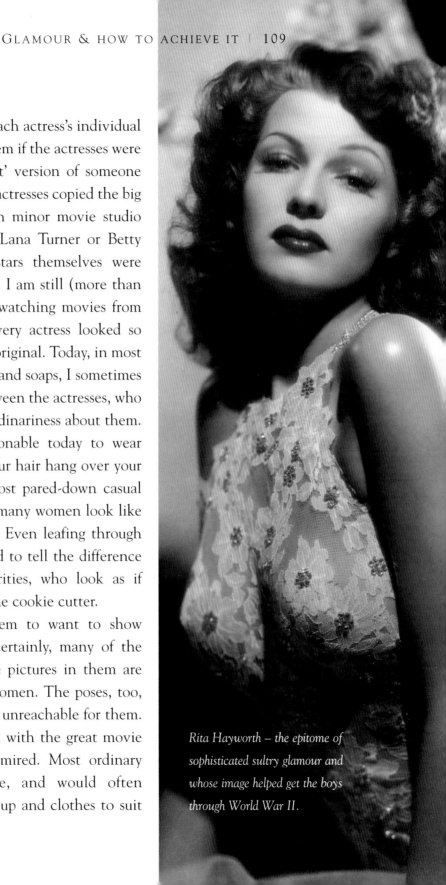

Rita Hayworth – the epitome of sophisticated sultry glamour and whose image helped get the boys through World War II.

themselves, for although these stars were special, in their own way they were also very *real* women that other women could identify with. My mother admired Greer Garson and Lana Turner and although she didn't model herself on them, she would often copy a dress or a hairdo, or the way Lana tied her scarf. Those stars were idols and icons. Innovative, unconventional and totally unique but they all had one thing in common: big-time glamour. Two of the all-time outstanding originals, Audrey Hepburn and Marilyn Monroe, are almost more popular today than when they were starring on the screen and are endlessly emulated.

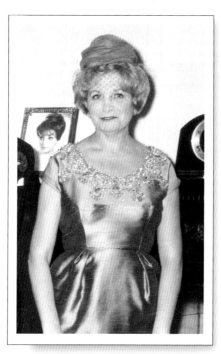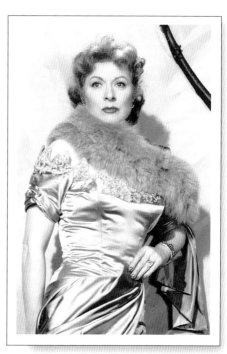

My mother Elsa (left) dressed for a wedding and looking very much like one of her favourite actresses, Greer Garson.

The life span of many of today's stars and celebrities also seems astonishingly short, which is not their fault. I could reel off (but won't) a whole list of big stars of the seventies, eighties and nineties whose names – and looks – most people would no longer remember. But how could anyone *ever* forget Greta Garbo, Betty Grable or Hedy

Lamarr? Along with hundreds of other luminous stars, their luscious images are etched indelibly in our minds and they all had the ability to raise the temperature of a room when they entered it.

I don't understand many of today's beautiful women and girls who, to me, seem to want to look plain. Some actresses appear to almost deride their beauty. I can think of several who are naturally beautiful but do everything to negate their looks. In paparazzi shots, their clothes look, to put it mildly, shabby and proletarian. Also, I don't understand women who knock their looks and put themselves down for being attractive. After all, beauty is a gift given to but a few and it seems wrong to be disrespectful of something that so many others strive for.

Throughout the 20th century, movies (and to a lesser extent, the theatre and television) gave the world an endless array of the most stunning women on the planet. Almost other worldly, their beauty was enhanced by expert lighting, the *crème de la crème* of costume designers and the most brilliant hairdressers and make-up experts. Some were not even true beauties in the strictest sense of the meaning, but their outstanding glamour made them icons.

From Clara Bow to Gloria Swanson in the twenties to Farrah Fawcett and Jacqueline Smith in the seventies, the parade of inspirationally gorgeous women was outstanding. But by the fifties, particularly in the theatre, being glamorous was passé and actresses like Joan Plowright and Eileen Atkins became the norm. Then, in the early nineties, with the demise of the supersoaps, among them *Dallas*, *Flamingo Road*, *Falcon Crest*, *Knots Landing* (and yes, *Dynasty*), glamour became obsolete and people talked about it almost as though it was a dirty word. However, I *know* that there are still a lot of women out there who admire glamour and would like to achieve it.

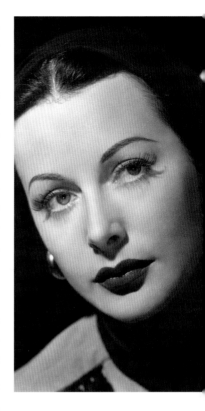

Hedy Lamarr, whom I believe to be the most beautiful film star ever to grace the screen.

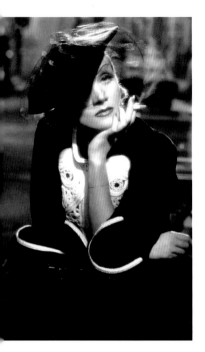

All-time icon, Marlene Dietrich. The most glamorous movie star, and one who knew everything about lighting and cosmetic enhancement.

CELEBRATE YOUR OWN GLAMOUR

Yet who can explain the true essence of glamour? My dictionary defines glamour as 'an alluring romantic attractiveness, one that is unreal'. I know that those close-ups of Marlene Dietrich, exquisitely lit and wearing veils, feathers and smoking a cigarette with supreme elegance, are far from the reality of today's harsh world, but there is something to be learned here, as from all of the other glamorous icons.

Remember, glamour is not necessarily beauty and it certainly isn't youthfulness. Dietrich was in no way classically beautiful but she knew how to make the absolute best of what assets she had. The same applies to Claudette Colbert and Katharine Hepburn. Dietrich's definition of glamour was, 'It's something indefinite, something inaccessible to normal women; an unreal paradise, desirable but basically out of reach.' Although her fans knew they couldn't duplicate her superstylish look, they adored Dietrich for her ability to look so utterly stunning, whether in men's clothes or exotic evening gowns.

MY TOP TIPS FOR GLAMOUR

For those of you who *do* aspire to a touch of old world or other worldly, elusive glamour, here's my advice:

Keep some mystery about you. Don't tell the world (or the woman next door) your innermost secrets. Be a little bit enigmatic, laid-back and cool. Men like that, too (even if they purport not to). And for God's sake, don't talk about your ailments, headaches or other aches and pains! If you're in pain, suffer in silence or take an aspirin and go to bed.

Become well groomed. No one can be glamorous with a hem hanging down, a run in their tights, dirty, down-at-heel shoes and dandruff on their shoulders. Make it second nature to always look the best you can. Even if you *think* you're overweight, be proud of your body. Make sure you have the right foundation garments or bra to make the most of your assets. Big breasts can look good if they're well supported (big droopy bosoms don't!).

Wear scent or perfumed body lotion, or use a shampoo with fragrance. Make it your signature, leave it in your wake. People will remember you. Scent is very powerful – and seductive, too.

Have well-manicured hands. Even if you don't have long red nails (usually a turn-off to most men) ragged cuticles and bitten nails are even more off-putting. So, if you must bite, keep them short and neat. Laugh a lot – men *like* women who laugh. But don't cackle or shriek like a banshee. It's un-cool, it's irritating and it's crass. Try to cultivate a laugh that's more like a caress.

Wear red lipstick. It's the most glamorous cosmetic that exists and also the most flattering. There are many different shades of red, from pale to dark, so there must be one to suit you. If you don't like red, wear pink or plum, or gloss. And if you don't like anything on your lips, poor you, you'll never be glamorous!

To those prepubescent in the late seventies, this picture should be familiar… (The Bitch, 1979)

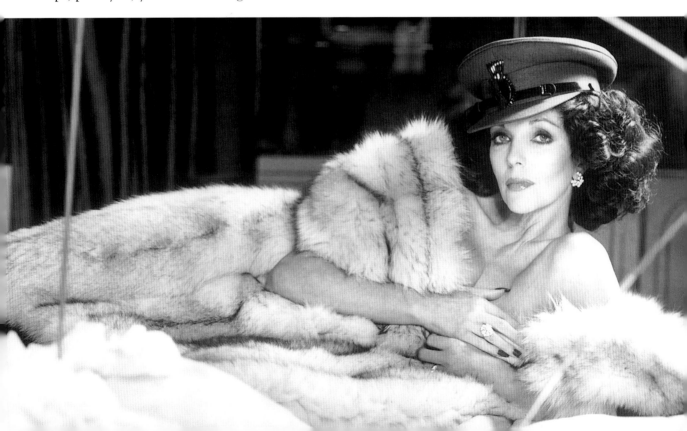

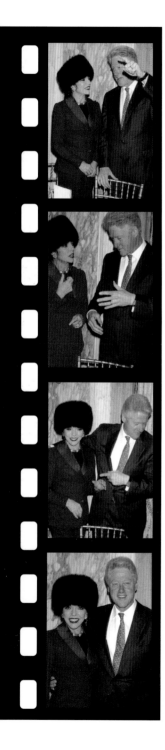

Walk properly. Don't slouch, shuffle, or stumble about. Keep your shoulders back, head up and stomach in. Try to glide. This is hard to do if you wear trainers or sneakers all the time. So this leads me to my list of the least glamorous of all clothing; these are trainers, sweat-pants, and baseball caps worn back to front. Not even Marlene would have looked good in those, although she did popularise extremely elegant men's-style suits.

Your clothes reflect who you are and what you think of yourself. Keep them clean, pressed, neat and tidy, and they don't have to cost a fortune either. Dress well. It doesn't have to be a chiffon cocktail gown – you can look just as good in well-cut trousers (pants) and a simple shirt.

Be individual: don't follow the pack. If everyone in your group wears their pants cut right down on the hips and showing their navel in front, *don't* do it unless you've a Britney Spears' stomach, which is unlikely if you're over 30 and haven't done 200 sit-ups every day. So know who you are – don't be a clone.

Be charming. As Sir James Barrie wrote in *What Every Woman Knows*, 'Charm is a sort of bloom on a woman. If you have it, you don't need anything else, and if you don't have it, it doesn't much matter what else you have.' You can get away with anything if you possess charm. I met Audrey Hepburn several times and was always overwhelmed, not only by her style, elegance and glamour, but also her niceness and her effortless charm. It was completely genuine and I saw her relate to everyone with the same intense interest. Has there ever been a more charming moment onscreen than when Audrey gazes at the handsome Cary Grant and asks, 'Do you know what's wrong with you?' 'What?' he barks. 'Nothing,' she beams with that glorious grin, 'absolutely nothing.'

Another person who has charm big-time is Bill Clinton. I've met him several times and not only is he tall and handsome but, as they say in *My Fair Lady*, he 'oozes charm from every pore'. At a lunch party at the Ritz recently he 'oiled himself around the floor' to my table to say hello and hug me. All the women at the table were knocked out by him, as was I, so I guess it helps to have sex appeal, too, when you're an ex-president!

And finally, you can be glamorous at any age. It is *not* the prerogative of the young. In fact, the self-confidence of experience is an added bonus. Some of my most glamorous friends are certainly not kids, but when they enter a room, all eyes swivel towards them.

Houston socialite Lynn Wyatt is always impeccably groomed and wears gorgeous clothes. Even by the swimming pool she's the height of style. Betsy Bloomingdale from LA and Nan Kempner from New York are both tall and slender and their high-fashion clothes are always immaculate, and the ex-Begum Aga Khan, who used to be Sally Croker Poole, has a timeless elegance plus the gorgeous cheekbones that transcend the years. These women *enjoy* being glamorous, whether in jeans or evening gowns, and that, I think, is the secret. You've got to want it to get it, and you've got to work at it to keep it.

Finally, one of the new generation of celebrities whom I think exemplifies glamour is Victoria Beckham (aka Posh Spice). She has her own distinctive, stylish look, *always* looks stunning, even when *schlepping* her toddler around or when pregnant. Of course she does have a super glamorous husband in our English football captain, David Beckham. I think these two young people have captured the imagination of the British public, not only because of their achievements but also because of their sheer unadulterated glamour, and I believe there are few couples today who can match them. I also think Catherine Zeta-Jones exudes old-time glamour and isn't ashamed of it as so many actresses seem to be.

One of the last of the great glamour queens is the legendary Elizabeth Taylor. I've known her since I first came to Hollywood when she was on husband number two and I had just divorced husband number one. I've met Elizabeth many times through the

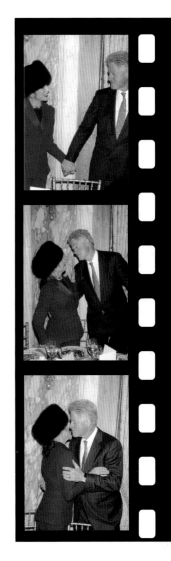

President Clinton trying to convince the author about what makes him so magnetic. He has charm but other attributes too. (London 2001)

Another great icon of glamour, Sophia Loren, with the author at Nolan Miller's birthday party (LA, 2001).

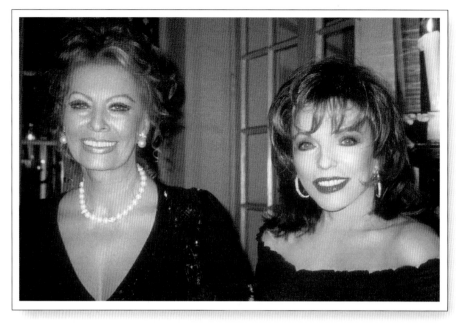

Opposite: Glamorous clothes needn't always cost a fortune. This chiffon animal print dress from Zara is an example of some reasonably priced evening wear. It cost less than $150. (However, I can't say the same for the bracelets and earrings.)

years and always marvelled at her incredible star aura. She has true glamour – and even when she gained weight and didn't look as good, she still had it.

Not so long ago I worked with her and two other 'icons', Shirley Maclaine and Debbie Reynolds, on the movie *These Old Broads* (a most unglamorous title with which we all had issue). The whole crew was totally in awe of 'Dame Elizabeth', as she now likes to be called. When we all did our first stills session together, the normally blasé technicians were completely riveted by her. Elizabeth exudes star quality and is the ultimate icon.

In the movie, Debbie, Shirley and I play three has-been movie stars making a television reunion special. To say we had fun was putting it mildly. The shoot was a riot of jokes, put-downs and gossip fests, even though most of the time we were working exceptionally hard and also rehearsing the tricky and lavish production numbers. Debbie and Shirley are, of course, seasoned 'hoofers', who've been singing and dancing all their professional lives. I was the novice and

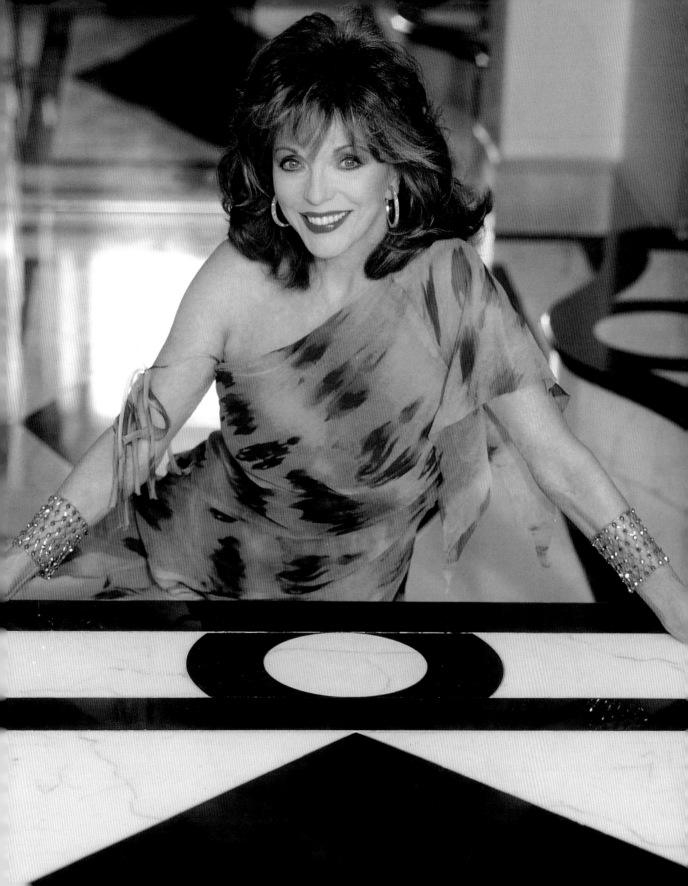

even though I have sung and danced in movies before, I was certainly not in their league, so I had to rehearse extra hard.

Our characters were firmly defined. In the script, written by Carrie Fisher (Debbie's real-life daughter), Debbie was happily married and running her own struggling Las Vegas Casino. Shirley was a dedicated but often out-of-work touring actress and I was an extremely rich 'gangster's moll', who flirted with all the guys and wore outrageously expensive and sexy costumes. This was a flamboyant role and for it, I needed to diet and exercise like mad as my tight costumes were extremely unforgiving and the camera adds ten pounds. I needed to drop eight, so I went on a really tough regime. I did over 250 sit-ups a day and practically lived on Wolfgang Puck's Chinese Chicken Salad (see page 54), which although you can only buy at Gelson's Supermarket in LA, is utterly delicious, easy to make and tremendously low-calorie. On the first day of shooting, I was down to fighting weight, thanks to my less than 1,000 calories a day diet.

'My God, Joanie, you look so gaunt,' gasped Shirley on the first day we worked together. She was eating an ice cream and handed me her cornet, 'Have some of my ice cream, you need to put on a few pounds.'

'No, thanks,' I replied, pushing it away. 'I daren't gain an ounce in these clothes.'

'But you're *too* thin,' she insisted. 'Your face won't look good on screen – you'll look haggard. *Eat*, woman, *eat!*'

'I'll ask Eric what he thinks,' I said and went over to our lighting cameraman. He almost fell off his chair with laughter when I told him. 'Stay the way you are,' he chuckled. 'You look terrific, on and off screen. I know how much you've worked to look like this, and it's paying off, honey.'

The following day Debbie asked Nolan Miller, the designer, why my costumes were so much better (and tighter) than hers and Shirley's. Nolan was forced to explain, 'In the script Joan's character is rich and you two aren't. Besides, Joanie had many fittings and discussions about her clothes, which you and Shirley didn't.' Which was indeed true. As soon as I was cast, Nolan and I had started going to the designer boutiques in St Tropez and Hollywood because I wanted to get the exact look that would be right for my role. It's what I did on *Dynasty* because I've always believed that clothes are an exceedingly important part of creating any character.

Nevertheless for a couple of days there was a certain amount of friction and perhaps just once the green-eyed monster *did* show his face. After one particular scene, in which I had just had an 'encounter' with my gangster lover, he unfortunately has a heart attack and dies. I had to wake up Shirley and Debbie, who were sleeping down the hall, to ask for help. I wore a tight red dress over the black basque I'd been wearing with my boyfriend, while Shirley was in men's green and red striped pyjamas and Debbie sported a pink 'shortie' nightie, bunny slippers and hair curlers. Needless to say, they were none too happy about how they measured up next to me in the red dress. After heated discussions with the producers and Nolan (which I wasn't allowed to be part of), I was put in a bathrobe in the next scene and they were suitably re-dressed. But luckily things calmed down after that and we all became friends.

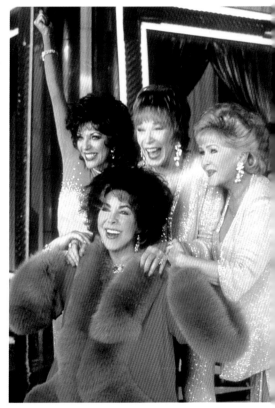

Four fabulous femmes feeling frisky. On the set of These Old Broads, *Hollywood 2000.*

Dame Elizabeth only worked three days, playing our agent, but she was a real trouper. She was truly in agony with a bad back and although she could hardly walk, in spite of this she still managed to look glamorous. During the scene when she watched us perform our final number, Elizabeth was done up to the nines in purple satin and matching furs, dripping with diamonds and looking fabulous. Which just goes to show that if you want it and you know how to do it, you can *still* be glamorous. There is, after all, nothing like a Dame!

Life's a bitch, so why not act like one...sometimes?

*G*ood gals finish last – it's sad but true. You must learn to assert yourself in life but unfortunately, all too often women who do assert themselves, and who stand up for their rights and say what they think, are called bitches while guys who do the same are respected for their toughness and strength of character. It's a sorry indictment of our times that strong women are characterised in this way. Frank Sinatra and Humphrey Bogart never pulled their punches, literally or figuratively, but just think how men and women alike respected them.

I won't be pushed around and this has made me a few enemies. I speak my mind and tell it how it is, and I *don't* suffer fools gladly. Unfortunately, the world has its fair share of fools, some of them working in the media, and as an actress and writer I often have to deal with them on a regular basis. Since many journalists class all actors as fools or megalomaniacs, why shouldn't I call the kettle black for a change? Sharon Stone once famously quipped, 'If you have a vagina

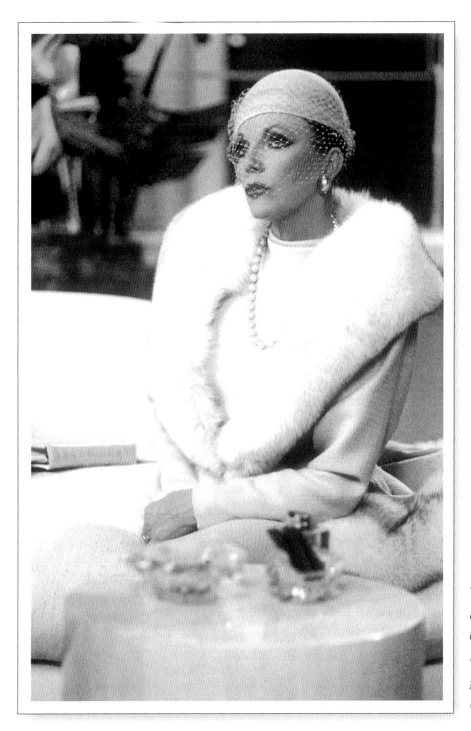

The bitchiest bitch of all, Alexis Carrington Colby, who always got what she wanted by fair means or foul. (Hollywood 1991)

and a point of view, that's a lethal combination.' Regrettably, women with strong opinions are not always popular.

Perhaps I'm not the most diplomatic person in the world but the dumb questions one is often asked at premieres and other events can boggle the mind. 'Why are you here tonight?' is a pathetic opening gambit, and not even the most seasoned interviewers leave this old chestnut out, so I usually come up with some banality such as, 'Oh, so-and-so's *such* a good friend of mine I couldn't miss his opening.' Or, 'I just *love* movies about people searching for apes in the jungle.' However, if you look less than enthralled by certain interviewers' questions they can sometimes take umbrage, proving they can dish it out but they can't take it.

Recently, when I went to accept *Maxim* magazine's Icon of the Year Award, I did some 'sound bites', which are short interviews. 'So, Joan, what does it feel like to be an icon?' was the question most asked by the folk holding the mikes. When I replied, rather amusingly I thought, that, 'It gets a bit musty down in them catacombs,' I received blank stares. At one point I raised my right hand to push back my hair and the reporter interviewing me squealed, 'Ooh, you look like you're gonna hit me.' I gave her a look and said, 'I don't bite, dear.' As I left, I heard her say *sotto voce* to a colleague, 'She's *really* a bitch.' I guess that's what comes of having a fierce reputation but I try not to let it bother me. Life is *not* always a bowl of cherries so I've adopted some strategies for coping with it and here are a few of the rules I like to live by:

BE ASSERTIVE

First of all, you just have to put behind you all the bitches and bastards who are going to call *you* a bitch, if you're not the sweet little good-as-gold girlie. As time goes by, dishing it out and not just taking it will make you feel better about your ability to cope with conflict.

Now this is what I call a work out!

It's a fact that power begets power. Allowing yourself to feel powerful enough *not* to let other people's opinions bother you can be one of the first steps towards becoming assertive.

You must believe in yourself and you must realise you just *can't* please everyone. There will always be people who will disapprove of you and knock you. After all, people criticised Mother Teresa and St Francis of Assisi, so don't think you're exempt. I've usually found that individuals whom people don't bother to be catty about are a touch on the dull side, anyway. Don't pussy-foot around, trying not to hurt someone's feelings because (a) you'll be doing it to your own detriment, and (b) you'll probably end up hurting their feelings anyway. Sometimes you may inadvertently rub someone up the wrong way, the same way others rub you the wrong way, but that's life, baby. You'll never be loved if you're too desperate to be liked . . . you wanted nunnery lessons? Wrong book!

SPEAK YOUR MIND

Say what you think and believe. Develop your own opinions. People may sometimes think you're a rude opinionated cow but you'll be amazed how many will really appreciate your witty repartee at parties or in the pub. Have you noticed that men can get away with the most outrageous opinions and beliefs? With them it's called 'discussion', but with women, it's often known as 'gossip' or 'bitchiness'.

It's important to keep yourself well informed. Current events, politics and religion are all fairly controversial subjects but if you bone up on them and have a point of view, you could become more interesting, though not necessarily more loveable – but that's another chapter.

At any gathering notice how people flock around an individual who has an opinion or something interesting to impart. You will soon develop your own little court in which you become Queen (or King)!

SAY 'NO' AND MEAN IT. DON'T BE MANIPULATED

Too many wimps say 'no' but don't mean it and they can be talked out of anything in a New York minute. Don't be coerced into doing what you don't want to do, whether it's going on a date with a drip, getting stuck with a bore at a party, or even having sex when you don't really want to. Of course some people may think you're impolite but so what? It's your life and talking to some old codger for an hour when you could be zeroing in on a likely lad is a waste of time.

Of course there are some obligations and events you can't say no to, even if you would like to. Familial or work-wise, we all have obligations and in these situations you should behave as well as you can. There are so many people who want to manipulate you to their own ways. For example, a boyfriend, husband or boss may attempt to manipulate you with logic (his), rules (his) and standards of right and wrong (his) to control you and your behaviour. Don't allow your personal insecurity to make him powerful enough to do this. (By the way, I'm not suggesting that all men want to manipulate women, but unfortunately there are too many who do.) If you disagree with his logic, rules and moral standards you are *not* at fault. No matter how much you may get called a stupid bitch or a stubborn idiot, *do not* buy into judgments or values you don't share. People who *truly* love you will give you the space to maintain your own beliefs and live your own life.

Salespersons in boutiques are masters of manipulation. *You* know the dress looks horrible on you, but she's doing the bossy boots act, and you end up buying the awful thing because you haven't been able to get a word in edgeways, then it sits in the back of your closet until Oxfam calls. You must appreciate yourself enough to say 'no' when you want to, to get that word in, even if you think you're being rude and not feel guilty about it, then or later. Guilt is the most useless emotion we can feel, and it probably was invented by bossy boutique salespersons.

TAKE CONTROL OF YOUR FINANCES

What a pity they don't teach money management at school. In fact, most schools don't teach nearly enough basic life skills. You must learn to understand money as soon as you start to count it. It's just too easy to leave it to your bank manager (or your father, husband or boyfriend). During one of my marriages I left all financial discussions and organisation to my then husband – not that I couldn't be bothered, there simply wasn't the time. I had two kids of school age plus a baby and I was working as an actress, too.

It was after we were separated that my brother discovered all the terrible things that had gone wrong with my finances. I *should* have found the time to check things out and it was a powerful lesson but one I learnt well. I also allowed 'business managers' to handle my

The ultimate nouveau riche bitch: Pearl Slaghoople in The Flintstones in Viva Rock Vegas *(Hollywood 2000).*

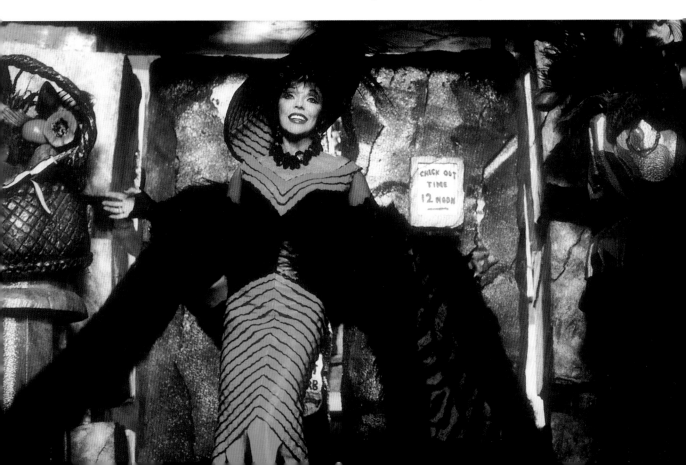

finances during the *Dynasty* years because I was working twelve- and fourteen-hour days. I became badly burned by that experience and ended up with a massive tax bill because my financial 'expert' at the time had 'forgotten' to pay my 1988 taxes. The taxman didn't care and the penalties and interest for that amount were so horrendous that from then on I vowed I would take (and keep) control of my finances as much as I could. And I have, in spite of the fact that I find it a boring chore. It has to be done.

It used to be that very few women understood the remotest thing about money. Many of my grandmother's generation couldn't even write a cheque and left everything financial to their men. Luckily, this has changed radically but there are still far too many women who don't take enough interest in their own money and how to handle it. There are many ways of getting a nest egg together. Even if you put just a small amount a week safely away you'll be amazed at how soon that adds up to enough to open a savings account, which can bring you a reasonable amount of interest on your money.

By the way, the money you put aside should be *yours*. Don't ever give it to your boyfriend or husband. They don't even need to know you have it. It adds a little mystery, too, and mystery has always intrigued men.

STRIVE FOR FINANCIAL INDEPENDENCE, SO EDUCATE YOURSELF ABOUT STOCK AND BOND MARKETS

It's *crucial* for women today to have financial know-how, and with so many women working I'm glad to say it's becoming much more common. Eventually you could make a foray into stocks and bonds but first, make sure you understand what you are doing. There are a lot of sharks out there in both the bull and bear markets. I know – I've been bitten by a few of them. So forewarned is forearmed. Force yourself to read the *Financial Times* or the *Wall Street Journal*. It can be boring but in the end beneficial. Ask questions of business savvy people, cull their opinions, then make up your own mind. Never forget that it's *your* money, so learn how to manage it.

Try to be as astute with your finances and business as shrewd businessmen are. Donald Trump once said that if he lost every cent he had, within a year he would have built himself up again to having a million dollars and in five years' time he'd be back to where he is now. I don't think we can all aspire to 'The Donald's' heights but we could all be cleverer about our finances. So start at the beginning: don't be reticent with your bank manager. Ask the bank how your money is working for *you* and not just making the bank richer. They may not like it but you have the right to do with your money what you will, and what's more to know what *they're* doing with it.

During one of my marriages my husband had gone to our bank without my knowledge and obtained a mandate in both our names that gave him the authority to sign on my account. The bank didn't question him and he had just given me a piece of paper to sign, along with several other things. At the time I was working very hard, getting up at 5.30 a.m. and not having much time for myself so I usually just signed everything he put in front of me. How stupid can you get? Well, I learnt my lesson when a year later, after we had separated, I found my account had been cleaned out. Although I went to the bank to protest, they showed me the mandate I had 'signed', so I had no recourse. Moral: Always read the small print on *anything* you sign and *never* sign papers unless you know what they are.

So don't try and 'please' your bank manager (unless you're applying for a huge mortgage). Your bank owes it to you to tell you what's happening with your money. If you don't understand, ask again. There are no stupid questions.

STAND UP FOR YOUR OWN RIGHTS

By this, I mean stand up and be counted, as an individual and as a woman. There are still a *lot* of MCPs (Male Chauvinist Pigs) out there who like nothing more than to denigrate or put down 'the little woman'. It's awfully sad that in the 21st century misogynists still exist, but fortunately younger men don't seem to suffer the same insecurities about women as the older generation (that's one of the reasons why I married one!).

My dear old gran imparting some wisdom: 'Always keep your face out of the sun, dear.' (Brighton beach, the thirties.)

I've often been told by some old geezer, 'Well, m'dear, you've done quite well for yourself with this acting lark. When are you going to give it up and live a normal life?' The cheek of it! I wouldn't *dream* of saying that to any man, least of all an actor. And I *do* live a normal life – well, at least it is for me!

BE YOURSELF

You are unique, one of a kind – be proud of that. But remember, life isn't a popularity contest and not everyone may like you even if you desperately want them to. My dear old grandma used to say, 'You can please some of the people all of the time and all of the people some of the time, but you can't please all of the people all of the time.' The important thing is to be yourself. Why should anyone like you if you don't like yourself? Remember to tell your kids they're great, too, but not to the extent that they become spoiled or big-headed. Kids need approbation but they must have discipline, too. Parenting isn't easy but it can be extremely rewarding.

BLOW YOUR OWN HORN

Some call it pushy – so what? The squeaky wheel gets the oil is an old truism. Job-wise, don't be pushed to the back of the queue. If you feel you need a raise or want a promotion, go for it, girl! They're not going to come to you and ask if you'd like more money or a better position (that'll be the day). *You* have to ask, and sometimes ask and ask again. Be proactive, take a look at what's happening around you and tell your boss, 'I can do that,' and why. Even the biggest stars auditioned, pushed and sold themselves for the parts they wanted.

If Marlon Brando, Frank Sinatra and many other great Hollywood stars can do it, so can you. After being the biggest star in the States, Sinatra auditioned for a role in *From Here to Eternity* when he was a has-been. The studio didn't want him but he pushed and pushed, and guess what? He got the part, won an Oscar and was back on top. It sounds easier than it is, but think of the line Sinatra sang in *Come Blow Your Horn*, 'Make like you're Mr Milktoast and you'll get shut out, make like you're Mr Meek and you'll get cut out, so go blow your horn.' And it works – try it. Sure, there could be many rejections but no one ever said good things come easy.

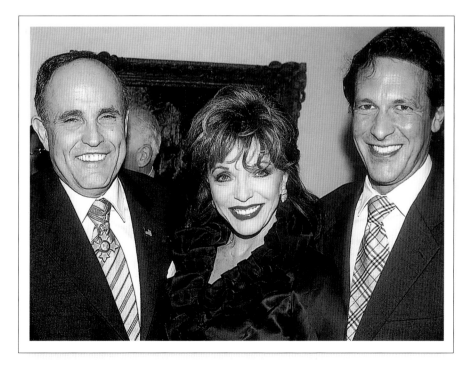

Thrilled at the opportunity to meet our hero. (The author and her husband at a dinner honouring former New York mayor, Rudolph Giuliani, London 2002.)

Dressing for yourself & your lifestyle

These days there's no such thing as the right way to dress. Practically anything goes, practically anywhere, be it trainers, sneakers, T-shirts with slogans, baggy pants, shapeless anoraks or baseball caps. I for one find that quite depressing because I like looking at well-dressed people. Watching people in the street is an eye-opener – so many look and dress alike that everyone seems identical. It may be the style of today but if that's *your* favourite guise, perhaps this is the wrong book (or chapter) for you.

I'm an individual so I don't want to look like everyone else, but I *do* want to look right for today's more laid-back world. As I've already mentioned, today much of the West suffers from a serious surfeit of youth mania and too many women of a certain age are buying into that craze by wearing totally unsuitable clothes, make-up (or lack of it) and casual

"You loved it on Joan Collins."

hairstyles. For example, long straight hair looks *awful* on most women over 35 and it also makes them all look alike.

Looking at a page of photos of celebrities recently, I found it difficult to tell them apart. The long 'rat's tailed' straight hair, the washed-out '*au naturelle*' make-up, the casual T-shirts and tie-waisted Capris or baggy jeans worn with navel-exposing T-shirts gives them all, in my opinion, exactly the same image. I myself don't understand the desire to look like everyone else. It gives the phrase 'fashion victim' new meaning.

Opposite: One of my favourite cartoons from The New Yorker *at the height of* Dynasty *mania.*

DRESS TO SUIT YOUR BODY

One of the major mistakes many women make is seeing a dress or suit in a magazine that looks fabulous on a 5'10", 112-pound model and putting it on their own 5'4", 140-pound body. It just doesn't work. Ninety-five per cent of the so-called 'fashion' in the style magazines looks farcical on anyone except the young and stick-thin. If your bosom is more than a 32b, forget it. A famous Italian designer of

Below: A gorgeous Maria Grachvogel gown which could also be worn as separates. (Claridge's, 2002)

svelte suits once said, 'I'm not interested in dressing women over 40, under 5'10", or anyone more than eight stone.' Needless to say, I haven't worn anything of his since.

As for older women (and yes, many fashion designers do class most women over 35 in this category), the average dress designer doesn't have this group in mind when designing. Many sketches for catwalk costumes feature a drawing of a stick-thin 6' transvestite with 4'-long legs, a 20" waist, 32" bosom and no hips. Many dress designers seem to deliberately show clothes that make even

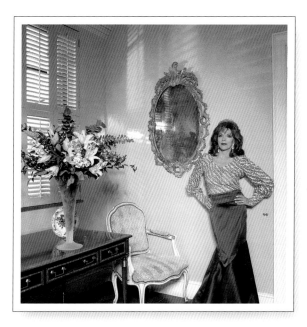

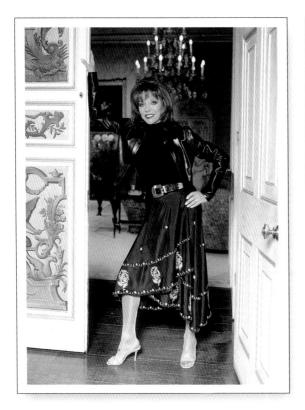
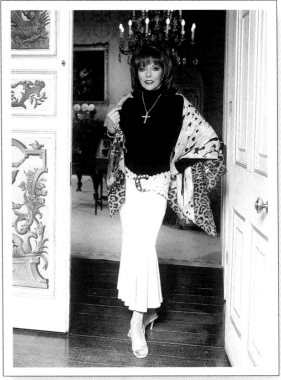

Every woman should have a black polo-necked sweater in her wardrobe. It's one of the most versatile of garments and can be worn with practically anything.

gaunt supermodels look either ludicrous or resembling $20 hookers. In *The Secret Life of Walter Mitty* Danny Kaye sang a song about a gay milliner called 'Anatole of Paris', who 'shrieks with chic' and whose 'Hat of the Week' caused 'six divorces, three runaway horses'. At the end of the song he asks, 'And why do I sew each new chapeau with a style that they look most grim in? Strictly between us, *entre nous*, I hate women.' That seems true of some of today's designers, but not all luckily.

It's ridiculous for a normal woman to even attempt to live up to the expectations of designers or to try and emulate the Giselle Bundchen generation of under-25s. Today model agents are looking for ever-younger girls to fill their books. My friend, Stella Wilson, has a beautiful seventeen-year-old daughter, Amy Thomas, who, since

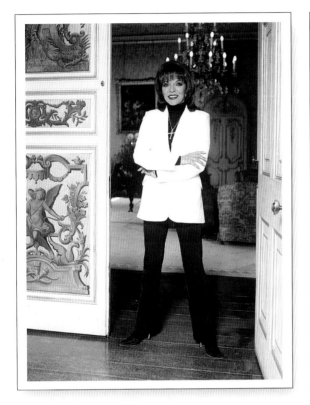
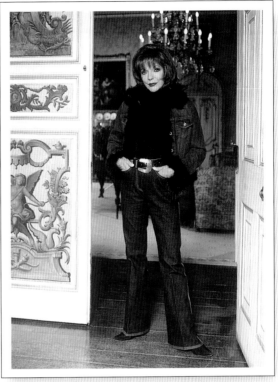

she was fourteen, has been stopped in the street by modelling talent scouts asking if she would like to become a model. Also Charles and Pandora Delevingne's two teenage daughters, Chloe and Poppy, have already posed for several magazine layouts, while their nine-year-old sister, Cara (my godchild) is *considering* it!

So how do today's skeletal celebrities stay so slim? The simple answer is that they diet like crazy to get into those slinky frocks that the designers lend them for awards and major events, and many of them have their own specialised diet cooks and daily trainers, too. It's a tough grind but they do it because competition is fierce in Hollywood – and, sadly perhaps, thin is still in. When I was on *Dynasty*, Linda Evans, Diahann Carroll, the other actresses and I were instructed to be at least eight or ten pounds less than our natural

Here, from left to right, I wear it with a black leather jacket and gypsy skirt, a three-quarter pencil skirt and scarf, a white jacket and black pants (two more essential items) and with jeans and a denim jacket.

weight, 'Otherwise you'll look fat on the screen', said the producers. And it was true – we did – so we had to eat less.

Once when I was travelling on a private plane from Paris to London, my friend Valentino asked me to deliver a huge dress box to Elle Macpherson. 'It's three gowns for her to choose from for the big party next week,' he explained. Lucky Elle, I thought, she's six feet tall and model-sized, and can wear with ease the most beautiful creations straight off the catwalk (unlike myself and most other women). Although I'm a British size six to eight from the waist down and have slim hips and legs, from the waist up I'm a ten or twelve because I have an extremely broad back and shoulders and a 36b bust. Since that is definitely not model size, I usually buy my own gala dresses or have them made. All too often in the newspapers you see ridiculous pictures of celebrities who have bought a trendy outfit pictured on a model and worn it themselves with utterly disastrous results, and the papers love printing those unflattering shots, too.

So here's some practical advice on how to appear your best sartorially, to look elegant and stylish yet not be a clone of the rest of the world; by the way, my suggestions for a basic wardrobe *don't* have to cost a fortune and will see you through most situations.

CREATE YOUR OWN STYLE

I'm a great believer in the separates look, particularly since I need to wear two completely different sizes. Separates work equally well at night and since dresses (with the exception of evening gowns) have not been in fashion for a long time, separates are the way to go and it's easy to get a look that will suit you.

So, how do you find your own particular and individual style? That depends on three things: your hair and skin colour, your lifestyle and your size. First, take a long, hard look at yourself in a three-way mirror (naked, if you can stand it). What are your best assets?

The classic white shirt, which can go with practically anything and always looks good. Here, with a jeans skirt and simple straw hat.

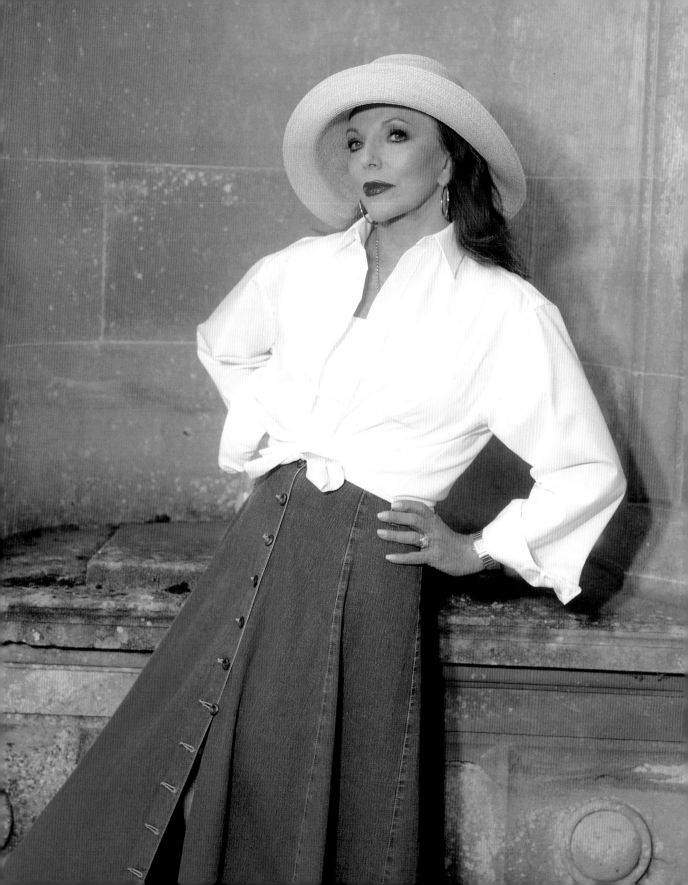

Everyone has them. If you are a touch overweight then perhaps you have really good skin, which is one of the advantages of being a little bit plump. In that case you should draw attention to the skin on your arms, or upper chest, or hands, by wearing clothes that enhance and display those assets. For example, you don't have to show masses of cleavage but the peasant and gypsy blouses in the high street stores now have drawstring necks that can show as much or as little skin as you wish. The forearms and hands on women over size 14 or 16 are usually excellent, so wearing three-quarter or elbow-length sleeves is flattering, as are rings and bracelets which look much better on a plump hand than a scrawny one. Bright, unusual nail colour draws attention to these as well.

I love this frilly blouse and it covers a multitude of sins if I've eaten too much.

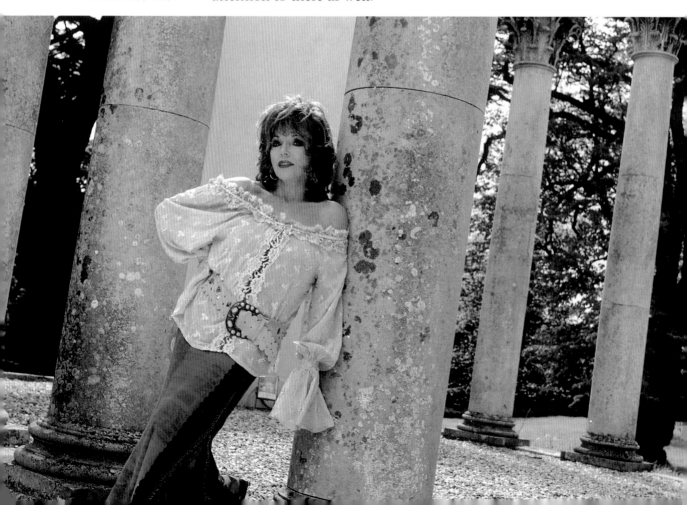

If your waist is thick, the peasant blouse is a godsend as it disguises a multitude of sins. And if you're too thin (although as socialite and forties *Vogue* fashion editor Babe Paley once said, 'You can never be too thin or too rich,') accentuating your waist can make even the most mundane outfit look stylish. A white tank top or shirt tucked into jeans or boot-cut pants looks great set off with a wide belt. And there are zillions to choose from now. Belts are back with a vengeance and if, like me, you've been hoarding a few at the back of your closet, bring them out again. They can tie lots of garments together for an up-to-date look.

If you're tall and heavy, the caftan or Muu Muu, out of favour fashion-wise since the seventies, has made a huge comeback – and there are many to choose from. Yves Saint Laurent did dozens, mostly in animal print silk or chiffon, and if you can do some simple sewing (or find a dressmaker), a trip to your nearest fabric store will yield a veritable Aladdin's cave of gorgeous fabrics to make up your own version.

I adore going fabric shopping and when I'm travelling I always try and buy lengths of material to have things made. On a recent trip to Malaysia I fell in love again with batik, which is translated as 'a cloth with little dots', and had some beautiful things made by my dressmaker (whose name I shan't reveal because I don't want her stolen from me as has happened in the past!).

If you have a big butt *please* don't wear tight jeans or Lycra shorts. Look at yourself in your three-way mirror, particularly the back view. Remember Dumbo? A long, loose thigh-length shirt or coat conceals a great deal and, worn over a simple T-shirt in a flattering colour, it can also do much to enhance the fuller figure. My friend, the actress Miriam Margolyes, describes herself as short, fat and 50, but dresses cleverly in bold prints and loose clothes so she almost makes an asset out of being only five feet tall. If you don't want to

Caftan, circa 1970s.

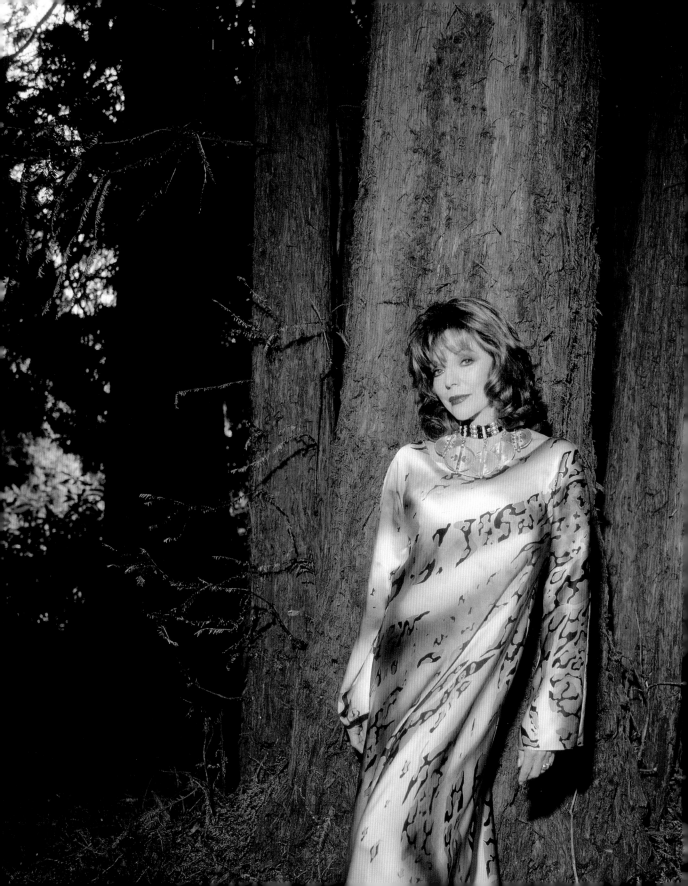

wear a full-length caftan, a shift dress, knee-length or mid-calf, is a classic look and it covers up *everything*. And finally, never wear polo necks or high necks if your bust is too big. Instead, off-the-shoulder tops for evening are really flattering for that figure problem, as are V-necks for day.

WHAT EVERY WOMAN SHOULD HAVE IN HER WARDROBE

This is a basic collection of only about twenty classic pieces, which may sound a lot if you're starting from scratch but you've probably got at least half of them in your closet already.

White shirt and jeans and white tank top, or T-shirt and boot-cut pants with either sandals for summer or boots for winter. (One should have at least two or three white shirts.)

Opposite: Caftan, circa 2002. Animal print batik silk from Malaysia. My dressmaker was inspired by Yves St Laurent.

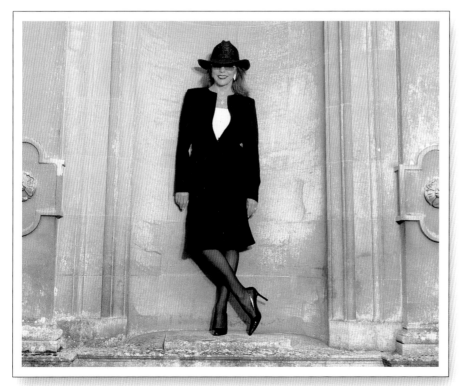

A classic black suit that can be worn in many different ways and is reasonably priced. (From Zara, about £130.)

I've always adored the gypsy–peasant look, and worn it even when it wasn't in fashion. So here it is again.

On top of this a jacket: one with the jeans (e.g. a jeans jacket is very trendy now) and then another one in tweed, black or grey.

Same jeans jacket worn with long black skirt and black tank top for evening.

Long skirt and off-the-shoulder top accessorised with different jewellery, scarves and belts for different looks for evening, i.e. this makes two or three looks by changing the basic outfit with accessories. Mid-length skirts (brown, black or grey) with jacket suitable for office, cocktail or every day.

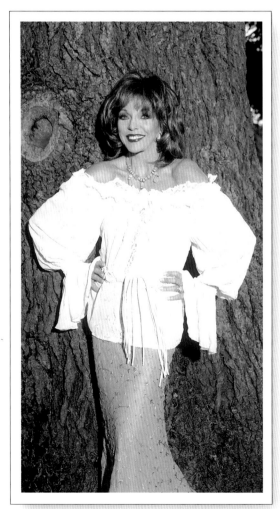

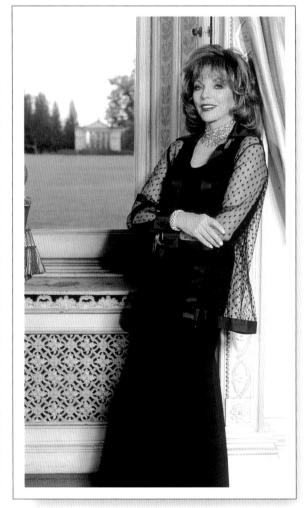

White shirt (same) worn open over bathing suit for summer (with hat and sunglasses maybe).

Same white shirt tied at waist and worn with long floral or batik skirt for summer look.

Long skirt and gypsy or peasant blouse for another summer variation.

Different variations of a black polo neck sweater with:

(a) Long black skirt   (b) Short black skirt

(c) Long floral skirt   (d) Black trousers (pants).

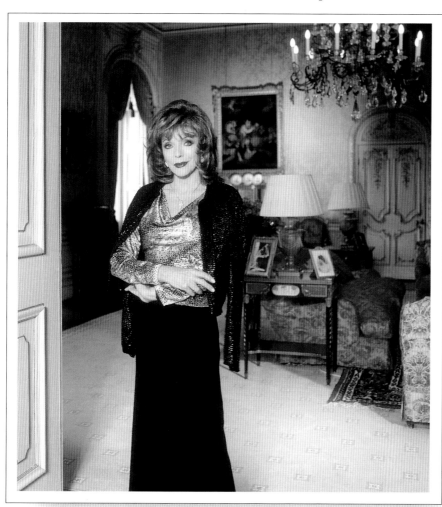

Left and opposite: The same long black skirt worn with different tops changes an evening look. The grey top is new and the Point d'Esprit shirt is vintage and has been in my wardrobe for fifteen years.

- One white pant suit with skirt.
- One black pant and suit skirt.
- A couple of extra lacy or sequin tops for evening.
- A couple of batik outfits including a caftan.

COLOURS TO SUIT YOUR COLOURING

If you have gone grey-haired or silvery white and have pale skin, bright colours can look wonderful. Brilliant reds and blues look great on this type, whereas black and grey drains the colour from your face. For blondes, white is always a winner, as are pastels. Intense reds and greens do not usually suit pale-skinned blondes. If you have a sallow skin, don't wear yellow (it's a helluva difficult colour for anyone to wear except for toddlers). Green doesn't suit olive complexions and brown complexions don't look good in brown, fawn or beige but again, bright colours can be flattering.

As I'm a brunette with fairly light coloured skin except in summer (yes, I tan – more about that later), I can wear black or white and also beautiful pastels like lavender, peach and pink. I tend to look harsh in bright reds, greens and royal blue so I usually avoid them. I also believe prints are terribly hard to wear (unless they're really subtle). I don't care what *Vogue* says, I won't be wearing any loud florals or those hideous mock seventies psychedelic prints that so many designers are pushing.

Whenever you buy something, think flattering not fashion. The garment should enhance you and not shriek, 'Look at me, I'm the latest style!' Heroin-chic is supposed to be passé, thank God, but it seems so many outfits photographed in the magazines expose new and daring, and *presumably* erogenous zones that are totally inappropriate for anything except perhaps really young things at parties and discos. Believe me, 99 per cent of women of any age don't look good showing a 'builder's crack' (or 'bottom cleavage') and few men really find it sexy.

The classic white pant suit – every woman should have one (I have six!). This one is by Zara and cost the princely sum of £120!

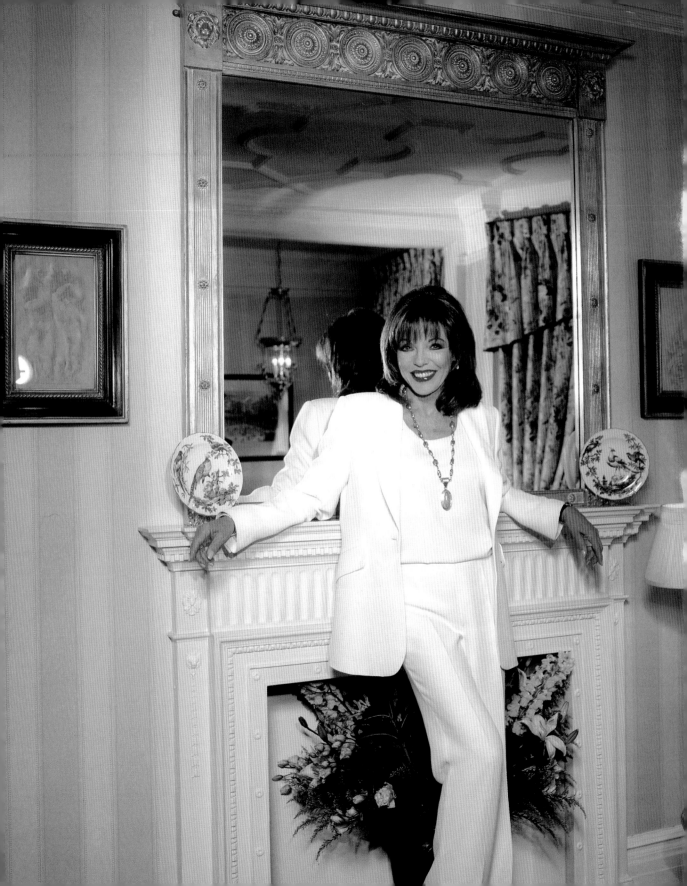

As for the much-hyped sales, with few exceptions, they are just that: hype. Most big department stores bring out all their old stock from the past several years and prices in Britain are still a rip-off. If you get to designer boutiques, such as Yves Saint Laurent or Ralph Lauren, early enough, and you're reasonably rich, you can still find bargains. Otherwise Zara, Marks & Spencer's and Bloomingdales do excellent copies of the top names that won't break your bank. I often shop there.

However, some sales, particularly in the States, do have fantastic bargains on classic pieces. Bloomingdales in New York is great for all things cashmere and in their sales they genuinely have a huge selection of sweaters and separates that are half the price of those in British high street stores. Saks Fifth Avenue, too, has really well-cut classic suits, pants and skirts, which are often hard to find in Britain as many manufacturers seem to think all women want to go around showing their navel. Wrong! Revealing that little hole is strictly the prerogative of the young and superskinny. *Nothing* is more unattractive than a roll of blubber hanging over the waistband of jeans and displaying a belly button, particularly with a ring stuck in it. It's bad enough on teenagers but on older women it's laughable.

SOME DO'S AND DON'TS FOR BEING WELL DRESSED

Coats should be classic and functional. Think Burberry raincoat and a long dark wool number. Your coat is an investment that should last a few years and it won't look good if it's the fad of the season. For example, I think that knee-length striped and belted coats will be extremely *passé* by next year.

Jewellery should be bold. Neat little pearls can add ten years. Right now ethnic jewellery is all the rage and if it's not too pricey, it can update a simple outfit. It's also easy to find as all the stores are doing it.

Wide, floating trousers are only good for wearing on a verandah with a cocktail in your hand. Pants should be sleek, not too wide and not too tight. They should *fit* and they should be long enough to cover your ankles. Above-ankle length looks awful.

You can't be chic if you're trying to look sexy. Too much cleavage and a too-short or split skirt may get the boys going, but it won't make you a style icon in your group.

Handbags can be a bore. You've got to carry one of course but overly

I love good costume jewellery and have loads of it. I mix it with the real thing, something Coco Chanel advocated.

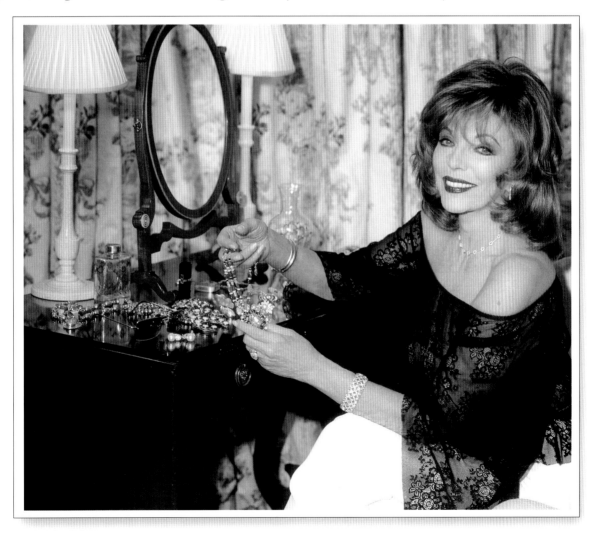

In the St Tropez sun daughter Tara follows my example and covers up. Her daughter, Miel, decides not to, preferring a cheeky look instead.
(St Tropez, 2001)

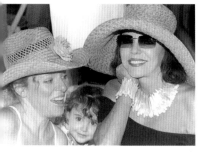

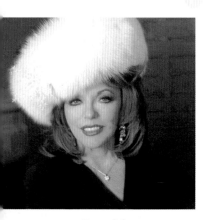

One of the more outrageous hats I was made to wear in These Old Broads.

expensive high-style bags are a rip-off. Have one or two basic shoulder- or handbags for daytime in which you carry all your junk and a couple of low-priced clutches to carry for evening. If you really want to look like our lovely Queen, carry your bag in the crook of your arm. (Why *does* she do that?)

Shoes. All women buy too many shoes. The classic court shoe or pump will never go out of style and it's good to have two pairs, one in a neutral colour (beige or tan) and one in black. There are a zillion gimmicky shoes in the shops but their shelf life is limited. You can't wear last season's purple python boots for long, but alligator pumps will last you for years, as will moccasins (which Princess Diana used to wear). As I have mentioned before, I have a particular aversion to trainers or sneakers, which I think look ghastly with anything except active sportswear or a nurse's uniform. I don't know one chic or well-dressed woman who would ever wear trainers with street clothes. Sandals in summer and boots in the winter are what I usually wear with practically everything.

Hats, veils and gloves can look chic and adorable and they add extra pizzazz to an outfit. I know proper hats and veils have been out in the wilderness for a while, but that shouldn't stop an original dresser from wearing one, at least in the evening occasionally. Veils, too, give the ultimate mysterious look.

Hats are great. I love them and have dozens. One of the reasons why I wear them is because even in winter I dislike the sun's rays on my face. Also, the right hat, even if it's just a simple beret, can make a look. Fedoras and 'Borsalinos' look terrific on most women. As for gloves, a pair of sleek black or brown leather gloves certainly completes a winter look, while long lacy gloves look really pretty with today's styles and you can find them in second-hand shops.

And lastly, vintage clothes are usually beautifully made, much better than modern (unless they're couture) and the advantage of vintage is that you'll be totally original, if that's what you want. Vintage can even be something just ten years old. I store a lot of things at the back of my closet (*yes*, I hoard) that look fabulous when I recycle them a few years later.

A pillbox hat with veil, which I might wear occasionally to a drinks party.

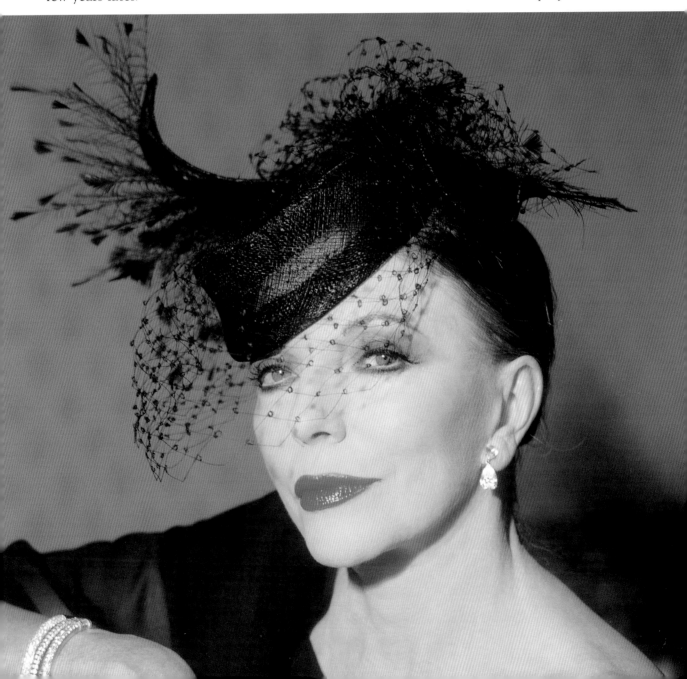

When life gives you lemons, make lemonade

I believe that there are really only two kinds of people in this world: winners and losers; survivors or those who go down with the ship. However, being a winner doesn't mean you have to be a company boss or run the most impeccable house on your street, and being a survivor doesn't mean treading water while you float towards dry land, however much this may sometimes be an accurate representation of life. Surviving is really an appreciation of life and what life is all about. Life is *not* a contest. There are so many things to appreciate in daily living that we take for granted, among them our own and our family's health, food and shelter, and a civilised place to live in.

It isn't by chance that many people over 50 look, feel and have more energy than many 30-year-olds. It's a conscious decision they've taken because they have learned it's all in their hands. Older people come from an era in which you got out of life what you put into it and they don't expect handouts. In the past there was no 'these are my rights' and 'I'm entitled to this' nonsense. People were expected to give to society if they were going to get something back from it which unfortunately, many people can't seem to comprehend. When William Ernest wrote, 'I am the master of my fate, I am the captain of my soul,' he was saying it like it is.

But everyone's life is a bit of a roller coaster. What goes up must come down, and whoever said life was a bed of roses was fooling themselves. The petals are there, but so are the thorns. Fortunately, I am an incurable optimist. To me the glass is always half-full, never half-empty, and I always try to see the best in everyone and most situations. So when life gives you lemons, which it undoubtedly will, try and make lemonade. From an early age I knew that the world was not a place where everyone lived happily ever after or where Prince

Alexis never let life get her down, even when faced with the naked hatred of Mr and Mrs Carrington (Dynasty, 1986).

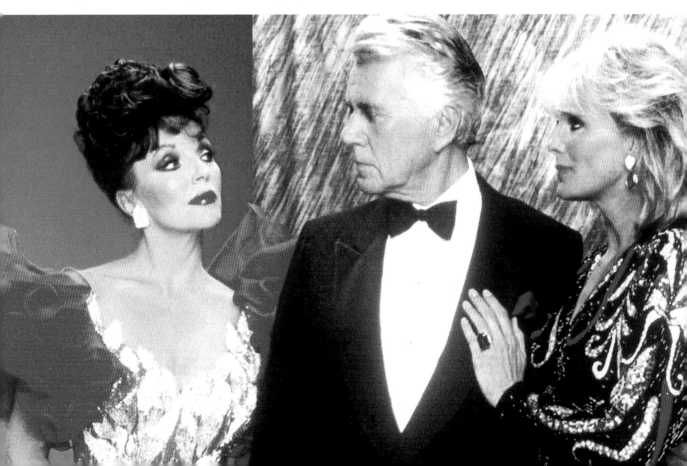

Charming existed. I think one of the reasons I have survived is because this knowledge has made me incredibly resilient and not neurotic. Well, considerably less neurotic than many actresses I know.

Even though things have not always been easy in my life, I'm aware of how lucky I really am and I get great joy from my life. But looking back on the *Dynasty* years, my life was, to say the least, troubled. My eight-year-old daughter was recovering from an accident, my father became sick and then died and my then husband started getting into heavy drugs. We divorced and soon after he, too, died. Not connected with this, my brother then discovered that all the money in my London bank account had been embezzled and I had to sell my London flat as I owed money to the bank. To top it all off, I married again and that *really* was one of the biggest mistakes of my life. My new husband proved himself to be not only an adulterer, but also a liar, to say the least. After less than a year of marriage I found the courage to divorce him and was delighted when the judge ruled both in my favour and that of the pre-nuptial agreement I had insisted on.

Now, you are either strong enough to live with all these knocks or you are not. I guess I was, because each right hook was closely followed by an uppercut, but I wouldn't allow myself to give in. I was the sole supporter of my three children, I was still paying for their education and I *had* to be strong for them. I told them I would help them as much as I could while they were growing up, but finally the ball must be in their court, and I admire them for what they have achieved because although they sometimes struggle, they are doing well and succeeding in *life*, which is the main thing that matters.

Just another day in a Diva's life! On location in the back streets of Los Angeles with (from left to right) Rene Horsch and Mark Zunnino (dress designers), Judy Bryer (my personal assistant), Andi Sidell (make-up artiste), Jeffrey Lane (publicist) and Gerald Solomon (hairdresser). Oh, the glamour of it – not! (Los Angeles, 2000)

It can be empowering to have good and bad experiences. The happiest people I know are those who battle through the lows in life because they know how high the heights can be. Consequently they have more of an appreciation of the value of life.

I've written in my autobiography, *Second Act*, about my harrowing court saga, a million-dollar battle screened against my will to millions of TV watchers, in which I vindicated myself

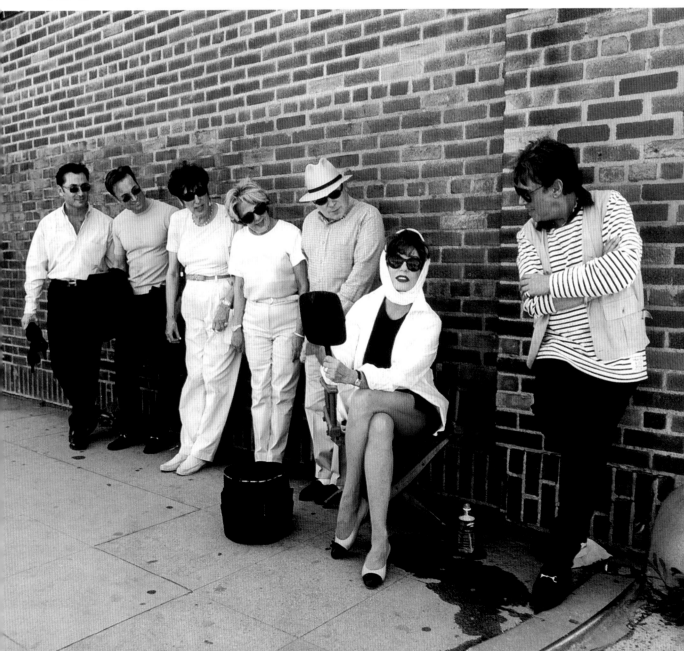

against one of the most powerful publishing houses in the world when my integrity as a writer was thrown into question. Most of the time I don't allow things to affect me; however a recent experience was quite unsettling to say the least. I've worked with hundreds of actors and actresses during my career and with extremely few exceptions they have all been agreeable, talented and industrious. Acting is a tough profession and you have to be extremely resilient to survive. You have to go with all the punches, which in some cases can even be body blows. There are no guarantees in the theatrical profession (which encompasses stage, film, concerts and television) and an individual has to be girded up for potential rejection at all times. For those misbegotten souls who believe that actors are nothing but a bunch of self-absorbed narcissists, I should like to set the record straight. On the whole, actors are the most hard-working, self-reliant and amicable people you could ever hope to meet. Most of them are witty and fun to be around, love their craft and would like to practise it more. However, it's the cruellest of professions and even the most worthy of actors seldom get the acclaim they deserve. The Brad Pitts and Julia Roberts of the acting world are very few and far between, and 95 per cent of us rarely know where our next job is coming from and whether we will be able to pay the mortgage this year.

To actually make a decent living in the acting profession is exceptional and to continue working for decades is a major miracle. I consider myself blessed and lucky to have done both but there have been many, many setbacks and rejections and on occasion, I've been saddled with a couple of truly difficult and temperamental actors.

One of the most unsettling experiences was with a big American movie star, whom I shall call 'Blondy'. Blondy gave new meaning to the word 'cocksure' and made no bones about his intentions towards little me. We were on location and I had my two toddlers in tow, plus a nanny. I considered myself fortunate to have the gig for, having recently turned the wrong side of 30, I was well aware that the sand was running out for my leading lady days. There were dozens of actresses all competing for the same roles, but I felt I had won this particular role over some stiff competition and although it wasn't an Oscar-winning role, it was a decent enough part opposite a major star. But everyone acted as if they were treading on eggshells around Blondy. I, however, have never been famous for my diplomacy so when Mr B made, to put it bluntly, an extremely obvious pass while we were together in my hotel room. I turned him down with that age-old excuse, 'Oh no, I can't. I'm married!' 'But he's in England,' persisted Blondy. 'He's coming out next week,' I gasped, evading his octopus clutches. 'We've still got time,' he drawled. 'No, no,' I said in my Victorian maiden's voice. 'There's someone else in my life, too.' 'What?' he looked shocked. 'Another guy?' 'Yes,' I said, meekly. 'So you see I couldn't possibly…' 'What difference can one more make then?' he grinned as he tried to launch himself upon me enthusiastically.

I fought him off, literally, until he got the picture and stumbled to the door. Turning to me, he hissed, 'You bitch! You've done it now.' 'What have I *done?*' I asked, indignantly. 'I just told you the truth.' 'Wait and see,' said Blondy ominously and slammed the door. His revenge for being turned down was to send me to Coventry for the rest of the shoot. He simply refused to talk to me at all, on or off the set. Only when we were shooting a scene would he speak to me and then only in character. It was exceedingly disconcerting, not to say upsetting to endure the next six weeks, but I was determined Blondy wasn't going to get me down and addressed remarks to him in front of the crew even though I knew he wouldn't acknowledge them. Although they wouldn't dare show it in front of him, the crew found this hilarious. In spite of my happy face, it was a horrible experience. The worst time was the love scene, which we shot on the last day, in which I was naked from the waist up. I had been dreading it but I just put my mind in another place. I pretended it wasn't me in front of the crew with the dreaded Blondy, who wanted to savour my embarrassment by making several chauvinistic cracks to them. I have never been so pleased as when the director called 'Cut and print' and I was free again. Free of the love scene, free of the dreadful chauvinistic actor and free of the sun-kissed island.

Some years ago I was appearing in an extremely physical play. I had a tough time, mainly because one of my colleagues who described himself as a 'method' actor, hurled himself around the stage with little consideration for any other actor who got in his way and kept altering his lines to suit himself.

Mr Method was tall and heavily built. My fellow actors watched him warily all the time since two of them had received sprains and cuts rehearsing fight scenes with him because he insisted on making them as realistic as possible. When he fought on stage he really went into combat with no holds barred and he was strong. One night he hit one of the other actresses on her head with his elbow so hard that he nearly knocked her out. The director begged M to hold back but needless to say he didn't.

In one scene M's character gets drunk and I had to shake and push him, pull him up by his shirt, pummel him and look like I'm rough horsing while his head lolled from side to side and sweat poured from his face and neck. Since I have some arthritis in my thumbs I had to be extremely careful and I had previously told M several times, 'Please don't grab too hard on my thumbs.' He replied mockingly, 'Oh, you're so delicate, you English rose – you.' After the opening night M started to further extemporise, padding out and changing his dialogue, and he became even more uncontrollable on stage. He insisted on doing things his way. He stepped on the other actors' lines and laughs and manhandled everyone in his 'drunk' scenes.

All we could do to protect ourselves was to try not to get too near to him which, when you're working together onstage, is ridiculous. I thought wistfully of a fight scene I had done with Robert Mitchum in *The Big Sleep*, in which he had to throw me over his shoulder onto a sofa, slap my face and then spank me hard. In every take Mitchum treated me as gently as a china doll and, although through the camera's lens it looked as if he was really roughing me up, he wasn't at all. To me, that is a *real* actor, one who's totally considerate towards his fellow actor, but who can make it look authentic while pretending.

One night during M's drunken scene when I was pulling his face round roughly to me, my hand inadvertently slipped on his sweat and I accidentally slapped him on the cheek. His eyes blazed and I was mortified and mouthed, 'I'm sorry.' In the interval I quickly scribbled an apologetic note, which I asked my dresser to give to him. But M didn't acknowledge my note and at curtain call when I asked him if he was okay, he glared at me and touched his cheek gingerly, which incidentally hadn't a mark on it.

Arriving at rehearsals the next day the director told me that M was furious because I hadn't apologised for slapping his face. 'But it was an accident,' I said, 'You know how I hate fighting... I would *never* hit anyone deliberately.' 'Well, he's really pissed off with you,' said the director, 'I'm going to tell the company that we've got to sort out a little problem so they should take a break.'

M, the director and I sat in the auditorium. 'So what's the problem?' I asked. M glared at me venomously and said, 'You hit me and it *hurt*.' I replied, 'I didn't do it deliberately. It was an accident, my hand slipped and I sent you a note after to apologise.' 'No,' he snarled, 'you should have apologised in *person*. You *slapped* my face, not once but twice.'

'Look at the *size* of you, M, you're 6 feet and Joan's 5 feet 5 inches, how could she *possibly* hurt you?' the director insisted, 'You're being ridiculous.' 'I don't give a shit what you say, she slapped my face and you slapped it twice,' he hissed, 'and you *didn't apologise enough*.'

I was so distressed by this ludicrous accusation that I burst into tears – highly unusual for me but being accused of deliberately hitting someone was a new and nasty experience. M looked at me and said contemptuously, 'Stop being such a fucking baby and stop bawling. Grow up, woman, and admit that you slapped me on purpose.' By now, to say that I was furious and upset would be putting it mildly. I ran to my dressing room to call my agent, who had already been informed by one of my colleagues that he'd never seen an actress treated so badly by an actor. The director then came in and begged me to have a rapprochement with M so we could keep the show running. I felt I had to. So I swallowed my pride, and apologised yet *again* to M and we then went through an uneasy truce. I found it extraordinary that *I* had to be careful not to hurt *him*, yet his massive elbows, arms and feet constantly flailed about dangerously. My agent came to see the show and said, 'It looks to me like you're frightened of him.' 'To be perfectly honest, I am,' I said, 'He's becoming uncontrollable.'

A week later one of the set doors became stuck shut when an actor slammed it on his exit. Stage doors are only made of plywood and are not as strong as the real thing. M immediately ran at the door and threw his weight against it several times. The other actor on stage and I looked on in horror as the entire set started to tremble. Then M broke the fourth wall entirely while saying to the audience, 'This is what happens in an ** production.' To say we were shocked was putting it mildly, but like good little troupers, we found a way to stumble back into the thread of the play after the set was fixed, and fortunately M decided to join us.

After two weeks two of the actors were barely speaking to M. I kept saying to myself, 'When you get lemons, make lemonade.' In spite of the fact that by now I knew M absolutely detested me, I tried. He not only seemed to be attempting to undermine my performance but everyone else's too and consequently, the play itself. He told one of the actors, 'If she *ever* touches me again I'm gonna throw her through the fucking wall.'

Weeks later during a scene when the whole cast are huddled on a tiny set, I had to pretend to hit another actress with my right arm while holding out my left arm for balance against a flat behind us. I suddenly felt crushing pain on my left hand, and turned to see M's enormous shoulder pinning it briefly against the flat because he had moved when he wasn't supposed to. My left thumb, which is quite delicate, felt as though it had been broken. Backstage, attempting to do the 30-second quick-change, difficult at the best of times, I screamed in pain. My thumb had received the full brunt of M's weight. I was trembling uncontrollably, in total agony, convinced it was broken, and I had to go through the last scene half-dressed as I couldn't do up the buttons on my suit.

After curtain call my dresser frantically came running up with an ice pack but since I was just about able to move my thumb, we decided it wasn't broken, bandaged it up tightly and I sailed off to a dinner party. 'I *won't* let that bastard get me down,' I muttered to a friend as I downed more wine than usual. 'That man is *not* going to break me.'

But the next day brought more bad news. The director couldn't keep the show running unless everyone took a salary cut.

Because I wanted the play to run, I agreed. I wanted everyone to stay employed (for some of the younger members, this was their big break). Everyone agreed to take cuts apart from M, who refused. Contractually he could walk if he took less salary so we'd *have* to close. It was pretty shattering for all the company to have worked so hard and have everything collapse because one actor apparently didn't give a damn about the other actors or the play.

Touched by the show of solidarity, the producer decided that the show would continue and that he'd pay full salary to M until he was able to replace him.

M continued to behave horribly, throwing in lines that weren't in the script and behaving so fiercely in the fight scenes that his fellow actors were black and blue. Towards the end of his tenure, I asked another actor whether he'd seen me slap M that night and he said, 'To tell you the truth, I didn't see you slap him at all. I just saw your hand slip when he moved his face.' 'Why didn't you tell me that, then?' I asked. 'Well, it was early days so I didn't want to make waves,' he confessed. I shrugged and, massaging my sore thumb, muttered again, 'Don't let the bastard get you down.'

A week before M was due to leave, I made my nightly exit with the line, 'Goodbye, I'm leaving you.' M immediately ran after me, grabbed me and dragged me forcibly back onstage, glibly extemporising, 'No, no, darling, you can't leave me... I love you. You can't.' It was a ghastly moment, the actor's nightmare, but luckily I wrenched my arm free, ad-libbed a line to the effect that I was definitely leaving and rushed offstage.

Backstage, five actors stared at me in goggle-eyed shock. 'That's probably one of the most unprofessional things that you can do to a fellow actor,' said one colleague grimly, 'We're not going to let him get away with that again.'

At curtain call M grinned, 'Did you like me dragging you back onstage?' 'No,' I said coldly, 'I didn't like it at all.' 'Good, then I'll do it again tomorrow,' he said malevolently. The next night, after the same exit, my supportive colleague stood backstage wearing dark glasses à la *Goodfellas*, holding a machine gun menacingly in M's direction, with several actors as witnesses. The method actor took one look at this tableau and obediently nipped back onstage. Everyone laughed and I realised that you had to try and give as good as you get with that sort of person.

One of the interesting parts of this absurd saga is that as soon as the problems began I developed a bad cold and a cough that stubbornly refused to go away. I truly believe it was my body rebelling against the non-stop stress. As much as I tried to release the tension and anger, it obviously still lingered inside me but as soon as another actor took over M's role I recovered, not to mention that my performance improved 100 per cent. As the saying goes, 'That which does not kill you makes you stronger.'

At the opposite end of the spectrum, in 1998 I started filming with that most charming, adorable and brilliant of actors, the late great Sir Nigel Hawthorne. *The Clandestine Marriage* was a glorious 18th-century period romp written by Nigel's partner, Trevor Bentham, directed by Christopher Miles and with an excellent cast including Timothy Spall, Natasha Little and Tom Hollander. I played the character role of the belligerent Mrs Heidelberg, complete with grey wig, blotchy make-up, red nose and yellow snaggle teeth, which were especially made for me.

However, after a couple of weeks filming in a beautiful 17th-century Gloucestershire mansion we discovered that our producers (I'll call them X and Y) hadn't yet received finance to pay either the

Dear Nigel Hawthorne in his red fright wig and me in my grey one on location for The Clandestine Marriage.

crew or the actors. Everyone was concerned and when Nigel and I asked our line producer what was happening, he announced, 'The bottom line is if we don't receive £800,000 by the end of today, this film will close.' Despairingly, he showed us piles of invoices and final demands from costumiers, caterers, wig-makers, prop, camera and

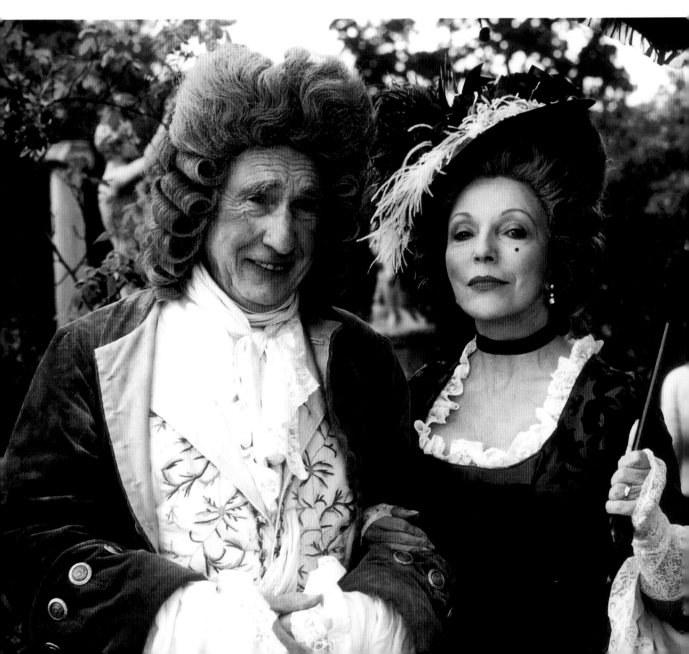

caravan rentals, and even food suppliers. 'It's a complete nightmare, everyone's screaming to be paid,' he added. 'Darling, this is far and away the worst situation I've ever been in, in a film,' said Nigel. 'Me, too,' I said gloomily, 'It's tragic that we're all so enthusiastic about this movie, but it's in such deep trouble it could sink faster than the Titanic.' 'We've got to do *something*,' said Nigel.

The next day our excellent producer, Tim Buxton, who found himself in the centre of a maelstrom not of his making, gave a sad little speech to everyone on the lawn, 'There's no money to give you, I'm afraid, but I hope that you will all have confidence to continue working while I try to raise the funding.' Complete outrage ensued. One of the crew yelled, 'I've got 25 pence in my pocket, how am I supposed to feed my family?' 'I'm very sorry,' replied the producer, 'but I'm doing all I can.' 'Tell that to my hungry kiddies,' bellowed the grip.

Work immediately stopped. It was absolute chaos. Some actors called their agents, who said that since they'd not been paid, they were under no obligation to work. One of the cast said he wanted to quit the film immediately but I persuaded him not to. Then the financial producers, X and Y, arrived and everyone trooped inside the house for another meeting. They agreed that they *had* guaranteed $8 million to make this film, but unfortunately it wouldn't arrive until 30th September and it was now only the 26th.

'YYY Films were supposed to have supplied the bridge financing,' said X. 'We've already given the film £200,000 so you shouldn't have started the film until *all* the money was in place.' 'They've got a point,' said Nigel grimly, the red curls from his wig blowing in the breeze. 'So why *did* we start the film?' yelled one guy. There was an uncomfortable silence. Our first AD (assistant director), Willy Wanda, gallantly took charge and persuaded everyone to stay. After two hours everyone unanimously decided they would stay until Wednesday but if the producers did not come up with the money by then, everyone would down tools and the film would fold. We felt utterly gutted. What was the solution?

I decided to do everything I could to try and raise some money and I frantically started ringing contacts in LA. I asked my bank manager whether the bank would be interested in taking on the mortgage on Mr X's flat for £300,000. Unfortunately as his flat was held in a foreign offshore company that proved impossible. I then spent Sunday on the phone talking to various money people and everyone else about how to save the film. Then my bank manager said that the bank would be prepared to lend *me* £300,000 but I would have to put up my house in the south of France as collateral. I didn't think that was such a great idea. I mean, I loved the film but I'm not insane.

The next day Trevor whispered that he and Nigel were raising £50,000 of their own money to pay the crew their per diems and to give them some kind of hardship money. This was so sweet and kind, but would they get it back? It was a horrible situation and yet everybody on the crew was being brilliant. To top it off, the news had hit the tabloids the day before ('Joan's film collapses'). My film! Wasn't Nigel in it, too?

At home that night, I called my agent Peter Charlesworth, 'How about if I put up some money? Nig and Trev have.' After he stopped spluttering he agreed it might be possible if the deal was done to my benefit. The next day we met at a restaurant with Peter, the producers, my bank manager and my lawyer, and it was finally hashed out that I would lend them £300,000. They were thrilled that I was making this 'gesture' but Peter insisted that I would have to get *my* money back as soon as X and Y's cash arrived. My friends thought I was completely mad, but so what? I believed in this film and I believed I should put my money where my mouth was.

The next day the crew assembled on the Gloucestershire lawn and Tim announced that a rescue package had been organised by Joan and Nigel and between us we'd raised £450,000. Then I stood up and, looking down at 60 rather miserable faces, said, 'I hope you realise that my money's good but I can't get it here from the bank until tomorrow, so please just be patient for 24 hours and I promise you'll all be paid.' Nigel joined me and told them what a wonderful crew they were and how good the film was, and everybody applauded and cheered us, which made me want to cry. Willy asked for a show of hands to see if the crew would agree to continue shooting. It was unanimous. Congratulations, smiles and hugs all around; it was extremely emotional. I rushed back to London to meet my banker and signed the papers for a huge loan. It was all a terrifying nightmare and I prayed the film would be worth it and I'd get my money back.

Five weeks later the funds came through. Nigel and I were paid back in full and we had enough money to finish the considerable amount of post-production. My fingers were now firmly crossed that the movie would turn out as well as we all hoped. But alas and alack, it was not to be. *The Clandestine Marriage* was not the hit we had hoped for, though it was by no means a failure. Although the actors received good reviews, the critics dismissed the movie as boring, even though most people I know who saw it liked it. Nigel worked so hard at re-cutting and re-editing and everyone gave it their best shot, but that's showbiz, folks. Onward and upward . . . at least I got to keep my yellow teeth!

Relationships, love & sex – everyone's favourite subject

Relationships, particularly sexual ones, are not just the prerogative of the young, although many of them believe they are, and are horrified when they realise that their parents, perhaps only in their late thirties or forties, are still making love. We live in a totally youth-obsessed society but unless we *encourage* people to continue all of the active physical pursuits they enjoyed in their youth, we are going to become a nation of geriatric invalids, not to mention a severe burden to society. Face this fact: most babies born today have a life expectation of perhaps 90 to 100 years. Should there be a cut-off date for physical love? Well, I don't think so.

I have friends of all ages, but I see an amazing youthfulness and vigour in them, *particularly* those over 60, who have never stopped being active, exercising their bodies and brains by dancing or writing, running businesses, playing cards, tennis, running, walking or swimming. This holds true for all physical pursuits including, of course, most folks' favourite: sex. Sex used to be about procreation, now it's about recreation. Use it or lose it – it works.

As you may have realised, I am a proponent of the theory that if you continue to do something you enjoy throughout your life, you won't find yourself with diminishing returns. In fact, as women get older and are no longer worried about the possibility of becoming pregnant, they can experience heights they could never have imagined when they were in their twenties.

Activity is the key to staying youthful in body, mind and spirit. Regular quality sex stimulates the release of endorphins, which are feel-good chemicals produced by the brain (chemicals contained in chocolate stimulate their release, too). It can make you feel and look terrific and energised, too. And here's some more good news: scientists at the University of Southern California believe that the skin patch method of providing hormone replacement therapy (HRT) can help women to revive libidos left flagging by the menopause. It's the older women's equivalent of Viagra!

LOVEMAKING THROUGHOUT THE AGES
Many of the most famous women in history have still been sexually active well into middle age and even later. Catherine the Great, who in 1762, aged 40, became Empress of Russia, was reputed up to an advanced age to take at least one or two lovers (and the odd horse) to her bed every night, and in her youth she had many more than that – lovers, that is! This apparently invigorated her greatly and contributed to a successful reign.

Mae West, who died close to 90, had a constant live-in lover, who was about 45 years younger than she was. She had much to say about the benefits of sex including: 'It's not the men in my life that count – it's the life in my men,' and, 'Too much of a good thing can be wonderful.' And my particular favourite, 'I feel like a million tonight but not all at the same time.'

Sarah Bernhardt, the greatest actress of her generation, had a voice that was likened to the 'silver sound of running water'. Her motto was, 'Life begets life. Energy creates energy. It is by spending oneself that one becomes rich.' Throughout her life she had a series of affairs with famous men, allegedly including the writer, Victor Hugo, and the Prince of Wales, the future Edward VII, and, at the age of 70, she even played Juliet onstage!

Sex is definitely one of the best and cheapest beauty treatments there is. Have you noticed how women in love usually have a glow about them? And it doesn't come from a jar, either. I'm not talking about tacky one-night stand sex, which although it might be temporarily thrilling, ultimately leaves a woman with that 'have I just

The glow that comes with childbirth. Half an hour after my first born, Tara, entered the world.

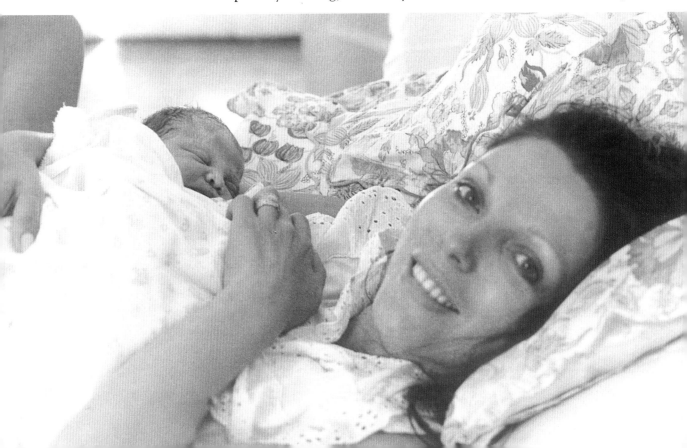

been used?' feeling. You don't necessarily have to be deeply in love to enjoy sex but you really should have confidence in, and trust and like your partner enough to enjoy the true intimacy that good sex can bring. After all, women *are* different from men as far as making love goes and however much they may try to deny it, most women prefer to have their sex life with one loving and giving partner. If a woman is lucky enough to have a partner who wants to give her as much pleasure as he's getting, then that's one lucky woman! You shouldn't be afraid to tell your partner what you like or don't like, and if he cares enough about you he will be willing to go along with your needs.

Atmosphere plays an extremely important role in lovemaking. Moonlight, candles and romantic music may all be the biggest clichés on the planet but they are often a stimulating turn-on that will get you in the mood for love.

Crazy for you… Five minutes after the author became Mrs Percy Gibson (London, 2002).

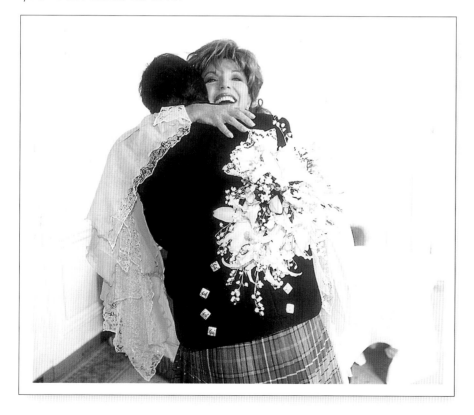

MORE THOUGHTS ON SEX

Most men, in particular those in their late teens and early twenties, like to have sex with a variety of partners, but unfortunately many young women today are trying to emulate their behaviour. Ultimately, this is extremely unsatisfying for women. I went through a short period when I was very young, in which I 'experimented' with several different partners (not at the same time, may I add!). And although at the time it seemed exciting, I realised in my heart of hearts that it was a one-way ticket to disappointment. Because I was brought up by the generation that considered it 'wrong' or 'dirty' for women to enjoy lovemaking; in my own way I was attempting to prove that notion was a fallacy.

Being in a relationship has always been important to me. I was far too young when I married for the first time at eighteen. It was a mistake that my subconscious knew at the time but in the fifties marriage was the desirable outcome for a girl and sex outside marriage was taboo. For most of my life I have either been married or involved in a relationship but I do believe strongly that unless these relationships are reasonably happy, there's no point in staying with them. I'd far rather be alone. Consequently I have been divorced four times. A marriage or relationship doesn't have to be perfect – nothing and no one is, and certainly not me. The sad fact is that people change radically practically every decade and often grow out of each other. Relationships aren't easy and they require a lot of work but they can be terrifically rewarding. I'm extremely happily married now and I hope we will be together for ever.

Strangely, it's only in most parts of the Western world that females seem less physically desirable as they age (at least to men in the West). However, to the French, *femmes* over fifty are still *fatales*. Our Gallic neighbours have long celebrated the allure of the older woman and the French cinema has produced a galaxy of beautiful actresses without the nubile bloom of youth but with a certain *je ne sais quoi* that comes with knowledge and experience.

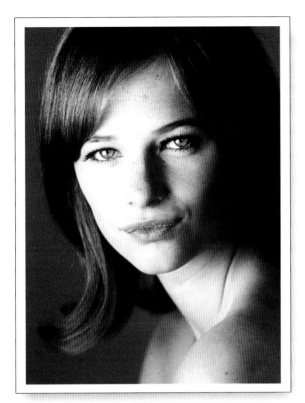
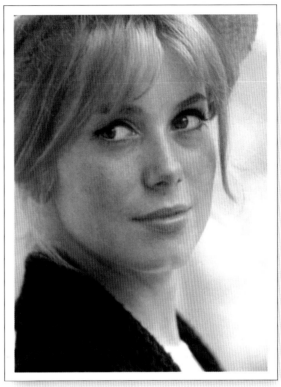

Catherine Deneuve and Charlotte Rampling are still gorgeous in their late fifties while at 70-something Jeanne Moreau is revered as an ageless icon. A recent study comparing American, British and Latin sexual behaviour reported that Latin men continue to find their women attractive as they age, as opposed to American men, who consider that only youthfulness can be sexy. Because of this, French women of a certain age ooze confidence and allure. They dress and act to suit their age while still looking soignée, sexy and well-groomed. Instead of trying to look like teenagers, they revel in their sophisticated maturity.

Much of the new wave of French movies celebrates the erotic charms of women of 50 and beyond, who are not tarted up to look like ingenués but instead display themselves in romantic situations with all the confidence of a 30-year-old. Hopefully, the time will come when

Charlotte Rampling (left) and Catherine Deneuve: Two superb examples of lovely women of un certain age. Interesting that it's mainly in France that they are appreciated.

American and English actresses are offered the same opportunity. At the moment we are used to seeing older actors, who don't look as good as their female contemporaries, romancing young girls. Remember Clint Eastwood and Rene Russo in *In the Line of Fire* and Woody Allen and Elizabeth Shue in *Deconstructing Harry*? And let's not forget Sean Connery and Catherine Zeta-Jones in *Entrapment*. But as for the older woman with a younger man in today's movies or TV – *quelle horreur!* That seems to be the last taboo, unless it's a joke like *Harold & Maude*.

I took a certain amount of flak when I announced that Percy Gibson and I were going to marry. As everyone knows, he is three decades younger than me, and before we 'came out', we thought long and hard about how our families (and the rest of the world) would react to our relationship. In the final analysis it was Percy who made the decision. He wanted to be with me forever and he didn't care a hoot what people would say. Being Latin, the age difference didn't matter to him at all. In fact, because I have enormous vitality and enthusiasm for life and all it has to offer, Percy often claims that I can wear *him* out.

Well, I don't know about that, but I do know that I've never been happier and more fulfilled in a relationship. As the actress Jeanne Moreau once said, 'Age does not protect you from love, but love, to some extent, protects you from age.' I'm not negating my other marriages and relationships but I remember that as soon as my babies came along (and mine came along *very* soon after my first marriages) things changed radically. Often women who have been loving and sexual throughout their marriage or relationship, and even during pregnancy, totally turn off sex after a baby arrives. I believe that's the way the female sex is programmed hormonally. I mean, if you still were as eager to make love a few weeks after your baby is born as you were on honeymoon, you would probably soon be pregnant again.

In Africa, Afghanistan and Nicaragua one sees teenaged girls who don't have the benefit of Western contraception with three or four children under the age of five. Much as I love babies, and I adored mine, that concept is anathema. In my experience, when you cuddle that helpless little mite your maternal feelings take precedence over your sexual ones. It's a sort of in-built pregnancy protector.

Just as young men are genetically programmed to be so full of testosterone that they are able to make love several times a day (and *want* to as well) so the female is programmed not to be so keen on the conjugal after giving birth. And because young men are so horny (there's no other word for it – sorry!), they will do whatever it takes to get sex. This means being lovey-dovey and sweet-talking a girl whom they may feel little towards other than the lure of lust. Many women, unfortunately, are suckers for sweet-talk and all too often are conned into a sexual liaison with a guy, believing it's love while for him, it's *just* sex.

Today it's perceived to be women's *right* to have sex as freely as men do, but I feel they are being let down. All too often young girls, who are reaching maturity earlier and earlier, *believe* a young man when he promises undying love, and jump into bed with him on the first date. Then they feel let down when he doesn't want to commit. Sadly, all too often the girl is left holding the baby, literally. This seems to be a teenage or early twenties phenomena, as most girls in their late twenties and thirties won't be so easily fooled, another advantage of getting older.

How things changed in the latter part of the twentieth century. The first fifty or sixty years was the era of good girls and bad girls, meaning girls who 'went all the way' and girls who wouldn't. The latter were regarded as the only ones who were marriage material because any female who was known to have had sex outside marriage was damaged goods and her chances of finding a good husband were pretty slim.

In the strait-laced moral climate of the post-war years, including the fifties, women had as their role models the pin-ups of the Second World War and glamorous movie stars of the time. But any hint of scandal would turn these same stars into box-office poison and finish their careers. When Ingrid Bergman gave birth to out-of-wedlock twins it ruined her career and although the studios used the beauteous sexuality of forties' and fifties' pin-ups like Rita Hayworth, Betty Grable and Lana Turner to entice audiences, those stars had to behave themselves in public.

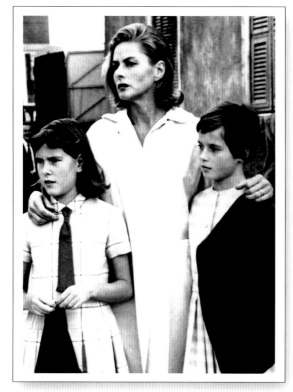

Ingrid Bergman, who was castigated and her career ruined when she gave birth to out-of-wedlock twins.

Although morals became quite free during the Second World War, in the post-war years women had to comport themselves as primly as Little Miss Muffet. In the late fifties America's sweethearts were a new breed of woman: Doris Day, Sandra Dee and Debbie Reynolds all epitomised the girl next door, the sweet little gal any guy would like to take home to mother. Then, in the sixties and seventies, women had access to the Pill, which gave them the freedom to behave as men had always done. Western women were finally out of the closet and accepted for the sexual beings they could be, and the seventies released a positive flood of books about female sexuality, while women's magazines trumpeted the new freedoms. *Cosmopolitan* was first on the bandwagon with its endless articles about how to have a better sex life. Strangely, its material seems to have changed little with the passing decades.

In the early sixties, when I was living with a relatively unknown actor named Warren Beatty, the Hollywood gossip columnists castigated me for 'living in sin'. Even though Warren and I were engaged, to cohabit was considered shocking behaviour in America, or anywhere else for that matter, and deep disapproval prevailed. Then in the seventies, it became almost the norm to live together before marriage. Nevertheless, despite my father's oft-quoted truism, 'Why buy the cake when you can have the slices for free?' people were still marrying, particularly if a baby was on the way.

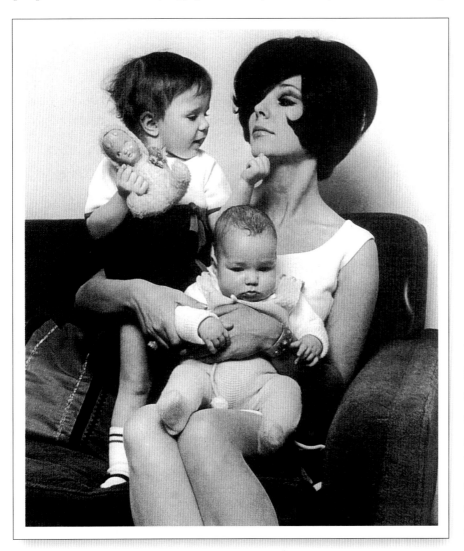

Trying to be the perfect parent while retaining my Vidal Sassoon coiffure – with Tara and Sacha in New York, the city that never sleeps, and neither did I with these two and no nanny.

I certainly made sure I had a gold ring when I found myself expecting my children.

Just as gay men came out of the closet in the sixties and seventies, by the early eighties lesbianism, too, had become not only acceptable but celebrated – today evinced by popular celebrities such as Rosie O'Donnell, KD Lang, Martina Navratilova, Melissa Etheridge and Ellen DeGeneres. By the mid-eighties, many beautiful and intelligent women were turning away from sex with men, preferring to be with women. In the twentieth century, women strove to have it all, but now that they had freedom, emancipation, and equality with men, they were beginning to find them sadly lacking in those qualities of sharing, commitment and the ability to love that they, as women, needed and, in fact, possessed.

WHY GIRLS TODAY DON'T ALWAYS GET THE GUYS

Today, now that women are able to enjoy the same sexual freedom as men, have they really gained so much? The women's magazines are full of articles such as 'how to have sex in the city', 'sexual thrill-seekers', or 'love and sex – what's the difference?' Today sex seems to be the driving force and unfortunately, not love.

While a big giggle for youth, the new 'ladette' culture doesn't inspire a grown man to want to share his life with a female who may, on a hot holiday, sleep with as many men as she can pull, drink until she's sick and flash her breasts in public for a laugh. The girls might get lots of sex, but at the end of the day (as they say), will they find someone who will want to be with them on a serious basis, or even marry them? And make no mistake, most women, whatever their age, really would like to be in a loving and committed relationship.

Photographs in fashion and women's magazines show models, although young and ravishing, dressed like prostitutes. Does this not give the message to impressionable girls: 'Wear this see-through mini-dress with a bare breast showing and you'll get all the sex you want'? Does today's man really *want* to see the woman with whom he is sharing his life dressed this way?

I first realised that I was attractive to men when I was fifteen and was asked on a date by the pimply-faced newsboy who sold magazines and papers at the corner shop. I was quite offended and told him he was cheeky. Fifteen-year-old girls of my generation were quite innocent then and as for me – well, I was still playing with dolls. Can you imagine a fifteen-year-old today saying that? She'd be laughed out of school.

I hope that sex isn't just what motivates today's woman. I hope that maybe the ladette-hooker culture we're seeing is just another phase in women's emancipation, like the twenties' flapper generation and the fifties' goodie two-shoes era. Because if that is all girls are seeking today, there are going to be some seriously unhappy females by the time they get to their 'sell-by-date'.

Perhaps there is something to be said for the restraints of the earlier part of the 20th century and maybe women today are pushing the envelope too far. Men often admit they want the woman in their life to be 'special'. What's special about flashing your breasts in Ibiza and drinking until you're sick? With all the freedom we have today, maybe women have lost something in the process? Or perhaps we just can't have it all? But we can try.

My husband and I as he skilfully tries to slip the engagement ring on my finger. (New York, 2001)

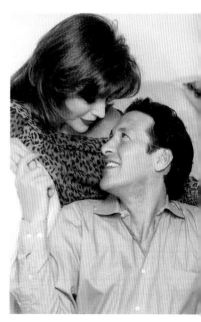

GET THE GUY YOU DESERVE

Sometimes your own insecurity about your looks and body can be a turn-off for your partner. It's important to love *yourself* first and if you do, he should love you back. And if he doesn't, then take a long hard look at this relationship and see if it's worth investing any more time in it. Often women are overly influenced by fashion magazines and film stars and think that's what men want *them* to look like. But it's not true. If he's the right man for you, it's your attitude and what's in your mind, heart and soul that makes him love you, not just your physical attributes. Physical attraction fades eventually, so it's the core of a true relationship that will keep your love going and growing, even though it was physical attraction that hooked him at first.

So how do you go about getting a great guy? It's not so easy. I have quite a few man-less girlfriends right now for whom it may not ever happen, but here are a few ideas for you:

Don't be looking too hard for a boyfriend and don't be needy – men are turned off by clingy and desperate women.

Play it cool. If you find someone you fancy, don't jump in the sack on the first, second or even third date. He will appreciate you more if he doesn't think you're 'easy'. Oh, it's *so* old-fashioned I know, but it's *so* true. Treat 'em mean, keep 'em keen. It works. But you *can* make promises and lure him on, be seductive without letting him seduce you. Men love the thrill of the hunt. It's true, they do!

Keep a touch of mystery. Don't spurt out your whole life history and/or past love stories right away, *particularly* the latter. Men don't want to know how many other guys you've slept with. Even if they realise you might have had a few, they don't want to think about it.

Become each other's best friend. Percy and I became good friends when we worked together and over the next eight or nine months our friendship continued and grew. Because we were so compatible on *every* level and liked doing the same things, later on we had a strong foundation for a really good relationship and a happy marriage. He's my soul mate and that's what you should aim to find. There are a lot of good men out there but they don't grow on trees, and are rarely found in nightclubs and bars. If you don't appear to be searching, he'll eventually show up. And don't just go for good looks. The best men are usually not the best looking or the most outgoing. Why not try a shy guy?

So now you've found him, how do you know he's the right one? Here are a few clues:

What's inside his head, heart and soul matters more to you than his looks. Sure, he may be cute but is he a fundamentally good, honest and decent man? Does he care about other people?

When you hear a love song, you know it's been written just for the two of you.

You have no doubts about this relationship. Your gut instinct tells you you're on the right track with him.

He doesn't blame others for things that go wrong and he doesn't point the finger at his parents for not being, or doing, the right thing by him.

He hardly ever criticises you but if he does, it's in a kind and constructive way. And he'll whisper, 'You've got spinach (or lipstick) on your teeth,' without embarrassing you in front of other people.

He gets angry or upset with people who are mean to you.

You love him even when he's asleep, snoring and unshaven.

He thinks your work and family are just as important as his.

He is *not* chauvinistic but he has a keen appreciation of other women, which is pretty healthy. Men lie if they say they don't notice or look at other girls. Of *course* they do. Don't you notice guys? If he's a red-blooded male he will admire a pretty girl on the street or in a magazine. As long as he prefers *you*, that's all that matters.

He has self-esteem and takes pride in his job, whatever it is.

He'll pitch in and do the dishes, and help with the grocery shopping and even cooking. He doesn't pull the 'I'm a man, this is too menial for me' act.

He takes care of, and organises his own laundry and cleaning, and doesn't expect you to wash his socks.

He loves being in contact with you. Hugging and kissing you for no reason other than he wants to be close to you. It's not a prelude to sex – it's showing his love in a warm and caring way.

He cares about his clothes but is in no way obsessive about his appearance. Once he's dressed, he's dressed. You'll never catch him glancing in a mirror for the rest of the day.

He likes most of your family and makes a real effort with them, and he adores his mother and sisters if he has them.

When you're making love, he cares just as much about your pleasure as his own.

He appreciates the little things in life like a new moon, a starburst or a rainbow, and crocuses blooming in spring.

He listens to you.

He laughs *with* you, not at you.

You can rely on him in an emergency. He's a 'take charge' guy – the one you want to be with if there's an emergency, a fire or an earthquake.

He likes watching you get dressed (and undressed!) and he *never* compares you to other women because he's a one-woman man.

He telephones you when he says he will.

He brings you flowers, even when it's not your birthday.

And, finally, every day he tells you he loves you.

I'm sure you can add to this list but here's another little list of reasons to realise he's *not* the one for you.

He cheats with other girls. It's okay to flirt but not to go the whole way, and he brags about his sexual conquests to anyone who'll listen, even you.

You can't count on him. He cancels dates and he lies, not just to you but to other people.

None of your friends can stand him.

He criticises you until he makes you feel insecure.

He can't pass a mirror without glancing in it and his favourite face is his, not yours. The song 'You're So Vain' was almost written for him.

He sulks if he doesn't get his own way.

He flies into a rage at the drop of a hat.

He hits you. Dump him *NOW*!

He blames everyone else for his problems.

He's too macho to wash the dishes, clean, cook or wash his clothes. And he won't even pick them up from the floor, either.

If he uses the phrase 'That's woman's work,' chuck him!

He talks too much about his ex-wife or girlfriends and sometimes slips up and calls you by another woman's name.

He berates you with your past mistakes and calls you stupid, and he insults you for having had other boyfriends.

He is extremely intolerant of anyone who doesn't share his views. He's also homophobic, racist and a misogynist. (What *are* you doing with him in any case?)

He's not interested in marriage, babies or a long-term commitment.

He hates his job and complains about it bitterly and constantly.

He doesn't listen to you – your opinions aren't important in his life.

During sex the only thing he cares about is how *he's* doing.

His friends are ghastly – beer-swilling, boring, arrogant and misogynistic. But he puts them before you. He'd rather have a night at the pub with them than a romantic candlelit supper at home with you.

He's only with you for sex. If you know that deep down already, admit it. Dump him!

He's got a drug or alcohol problem. This is a big No, No and leads to abuse. Don't be his babysitter when he's in the throes of addiction or be expected to clean up after him. Dump him *pronto*!

You feel empty inside and you *KNOW* deep down he's *NOT* the *ONE*.

Be patient. Better to wait for Mr Right than spend useless years with Señor Wrong. Give him the old heave ho. Goodbye Baby and Amen.

Thoughts on lifestyle & travel

My surroundings have always been important to me. I'm quite aesthetic and to live without an 'easy on the eye' ambience makes me less than happy. Flowers, cushions, scented candles and pictures of my family and friends in silver frames are all essential things that I use to make my environment more comfortable. In all the homes that I've lived in, I've always stressed comfort, cosiness and charm, which will enhance my surroundings. For example, I would never have a hard, dark-coloured armchair or leather sofa in my sitting room, however *à la mode* that sofa may be. There's no way a leather sofa is comfortable. (The same goes for leather seats on planes. I always put a blanket on mine.)

By the same token, soft indirect lighting is essential except in places where I'm going to be reading, putting on make-up, or doing my hair. As I've said before, for that I want strong direct lights, in which you can see everything clearly. Comfort is a great priority for me and everything in my living space reflects that. On my bed I have masses of pillows of different shapes and firmness. I love to watch television in bed and use the pillows to prop myself up for maximum snugness. My sheets are of fine cotton (I find linen too harsh), and the older, the better. The more often cotton sheets are washed, the softer they become but they must be good quality in the first place. Two cashmere or basket weave blankets and a fluffy duvet are also essential and I like a really big bedside table on which to have all the things I need. I also like to have breakfast in bed at weekends – it's a luxury and although I don't usually eat breakfast, when my husband brings it to me, I can't resist. I also make telephone calls and read in bed so one of the harder cushions props up the book.

When I'm on location I'm often lodged by the movie or TV company in a less than glamorous motel or hotel room. Since I bring my supply of cushions and candles, I can swiftly transform it into a cosy place where I can feel comfortable. I put different light bulbs in the lamps (some softer, some brighter), move the furniture around to suit my needs and drape shawls or scarves over the more unsightly lamps or furniture. I do this in the tiniest of dressing rooms, too. Contrary to what people think, the dressing rooms in both theatres and movie studios are the size of hat boxes and extremely utilitarian so I try to do a little magical transformation which makes me feel much more centred. I can't stand ugly furniture or bric-à-brac so I put other people's stuff away and arrange my own special things, such as candles, cards, flowers, photos and books. You'd be amazed at the difference it makes.

Whenever I'm on tour in a play and friends come backstage to visit me, they often say, 'What a great dressing room you have – it's so cosy.' 'You should see how it *really* looks,' I tell them.

MY TRAVEL TIPS

I travel all the time, crossing the Atlantic, making at least eight trips a year. I've also gone to Australia and the Far East so I'm quite an expert on this subject.

Here are my essential 'survival' guidelines and what I think it is important to have in your carry-on hand luggage:

A good book for the inevitable waiting. I always take one plus loads of magazines to make the trip go faster.

A bottle of water. It's important to hydrate yourself, and I often ask for water on a plane and find they only have fizzy or tap water.

Chewing gum or mints in case you feel queasy during turbulance.

A pashmina, or a little rug or throw to keep yourself warm.

Comfortable shoes or ones you can remove easily, and thick socks to put on if they don't supply them.

Dress in layers. It can become boiling hot or freezing cold on long-distance flights, so you can take off, or put on layers as necessary.

Dress well. In these days of heightened security, the more civilised you look, the less chance there is of a full body search, which can be seriously embarrassing!

If it's a really long-haul flight, take a tracksuit or a pair of pyjamas. Only in first class do some airlines supply sleepwear.

If you're going to the tropics, prepare for mosquitoes. For a week before travelling, take a daily dose of 100mg of vitamin B1. This subtly changes your body odour so that it loses its attraction for bugs. You can also sprinkle a few drops of lavender oil on your pillow to keep them away – they loathe the smell. Apply it to bites and stings, too.

Take your vanity case or toilet bag in your carry-on hand luggage, plus a change of clothes in case your luggage is lost or the plane is delayed.

Take cards or Travel Scrabble if you're travelling with a partner.

If you're travelling with small children make sure they're entertained (and keep them well behaved). There's nothing so irritating on a flight as a screaming kid. When I used to travel with my tots I went to the dime store (it's not a dime store any more) and bought lots of cheap cuddly toys and other playthings. I wrapped these up and gave them to the kids every hour or so. It really worked – my children were extremely well behaved and I used to get compliments from flight attendants and other travellers about how good they were.

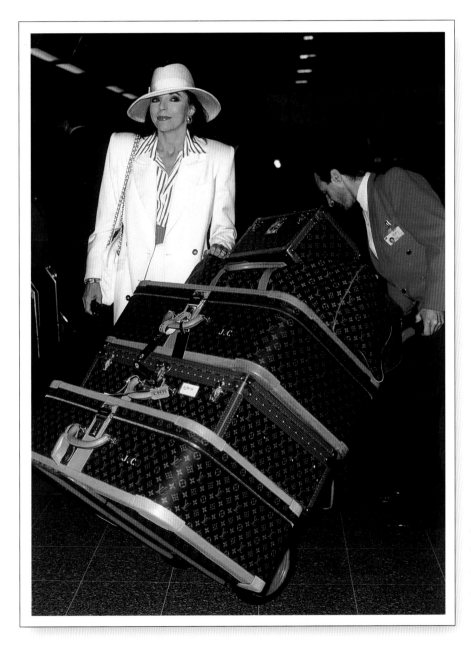

As many people may know, I've never believed in travelling light.
(Heathrow airport, 1987)

The art of entertainment

What image does the word 'entertainment' conjure up for you? A glitzy Vegas show, an afternoon with a soap opera, or perhaps a movie with popcorn and Coke? Of course they're all fun, but the most important image 'entertaining' conjures up for me is being with my friends and enjoying one another's company, giving myself to them and giving them the intimate pleasure of sharing my surroundings.

I have thrown many, many parties in my life, ranging from children's birthday parties, Christmas parties, twenty-first birthday parties, beach parties, pool parties, barbecues, cocktail parties, sit-down dinners for ten, kitchen suppers for four, buffet dinners for 50 and, of course, weddings – at which now, of course, I'm an expert. (And you must forgive me if I write at length about my own recent wedding, since it was the best day I've ever had!)

THE ART OF ENTERTAINMENT | 185

WEDDINGS INCLUDING OUR WEDDING

So, let's start with weddings. Whether you're the bride, the mother of the bride, the grandmother or sister of the bride, it should be one of the most memorable days of your life. For the bride, of course, it should be *the* most memorable. My wedding day certainly was, and that's because I wanted to remember it in every single detail as Percy and I *planned* and *organised* it with scrupulous accuracy. Percy and I had known each other for only twenty months, having met when I was touring in the States and he was the company manager. We became great friends for nine months, then the friendship changed and we fell in love. Although I'm neither a believer, nor a non-believer in an afterlife, when my friend, Arlene Dahl, who is an astrologer, told us that we had 'known each other in a previous life and had unfinished business together', it seemed to make sense: we had such a powerful affinity for each other. We felt as if we'd known each other before.

We wanted to get married and it was totally mutual because in spite of having done it before, I still really believe in marriage as the ultimate commitment when two people love each other. Marriage is also the ultimate risk or gamble but we felt so strongly that we wanted to do it. Percy had also been married before but, like me, he hadn't had a proper formal wedding. I wanted our marriage to be totally special and to this end, we decided to pull out all the stops and make it absolutely the best wedding day anyone could have.

We decided to get married three months before we actually told our families and friends. Remember the old adage, two can keep a secret only if one is dead? Well, it's true. Even if you trust your best friend implicitly, news of upcoming nuptials will race around the work place faster than Superman can fly. You'll then be asked a thousand questions, including: When is it? Where is it? What are you going to wear? Where's the honeymoon? Unless you want to sound dumb, it's best to have sorted all this out at length with your future husband so you have all the answers.

If you can afford it, a wedding planner (and *not* one like Martin Short in *Father of the Bride*) is invaluable. Siobhan Craven-Robbins, who was ours, helped us tremendously. Officially announce your engagement by first telling your nearest and dearest. Some couples hold a party to announce it, as it really *is* a thrilling reason for everyone to celebrate. Some couples' parents often like to put an announcement in a local or national newspaper, which is an excellent way to let everyone know at once. Of course, if you're a celebrity it will cost you nothing to have the news splashed across the tabloids. We told friends and family two months before our wedding at my annual Christmas party and the news was on the street the next day!

The couple usually choose the engagement ring together. With all due respect to your suitor's taste, there's nothing worse than letting him choose it and having it turn out to be a real dog. Remember, the idea is that you will wear your engagement ring forever so you had better love it a lot. Furthermore, hurting his feelings by telling him you don't like what he's obviously chosen with enormous care is perhaps not the best first step down the aisle, is it? After we visited endless jewellers looking at countless heart-shaped solitaires (all pretty much the same), quite by chance Percy found the most exquisite estate piece – a 19th-century heart-shaped cluster diamond ring set in yellow gold – at Fred Leighton, the New York jewellers. We looked at each other and immediately knew it was the one for me, as there would never be another one like it again. I love and treasure my ring and I wear it all the time.

As for the wedding rings, again these should be chosen together. In Britain it's becoming less and less common for the man not to wear a ring after the marriage. Because he's a dear friend, we went to the jeweller Theo Fennel and when we described exactly what we wanted, Theo insisted on us making several visits to see the rings' development and to have fittings. Your jeweller should take equal care of you (if not necessarily to the degree that Theo cared for us – he was a friend, after all). It's quite a sweet idea to choose your birthstone for a ring. Each month has its own lovely stone and it's supposed to be lucky, too. Finally, after your rings have been made or chosen and you're happy with the way they look and fit, you can each get to choose (without the other knowing) an inscription to go on the back of each other's ring.

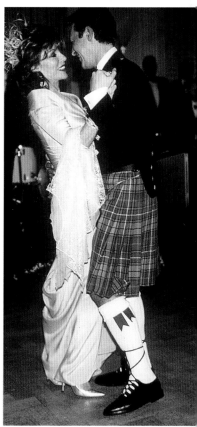

My new husband and I dance for joy at our wedding.

When you are choosing the wedding venue remember that many churches are often booked up months in advance, so you need to coordinate this with where the reception will be held, for example, a nearby hotel or restaurant, since they too could be booked. This is where a wedding planner is *invaluable* as the venue requires skilful coordination. Here are some useful questions: Is the place close enough? Can it handle all the guests? Will it provide the service and carry off the theme of your wedding properly?

If you have opted for a civil ceremony, either at a registry office or another venue, remember that it must have a licence to marry people (most hotels *do*) and it's necessary to book the registrar *at least* three weeks in advance (we booked two months in advance). The ideal amount of time to plan a big wedding is six months, but if you want to do it sooner, why not? We started planning our London wedding with Siobhan in mid-November, we announced it on 17 December and we were married on 17 February. That is a very short lead in to a relatively big wedding, which we organised and planned intensely, but with great joy.

We liked the idea of having the whole event at Claridge's

because it would protect us from the press. That way, we could have the ceremony, reception, dinner and dancing at the same place, but unfortunately this also meant we were limited as to the number of guests. Our original list contained over 300 people, but because of space constraints we had to cut it down to 180. This was rather upsetting to several of our acquaintances, but not nearly as upsetting as it was for us when two guests who had accepted didn't show up at all, leaving two empty seats next to Cilla Black, of all people. Siobhan said it's extremely rare for guests to do this but it sometimes happens. So be prepared for no-shows and, of course, people who cancel at the last minute because of illness, etc. To avoid any embarrassing situations, the bride (or groom, should he wish to take on the responsibility) should plan to spend the morning of the reception checking final placement and making any necessary changes. The wedding coordinator or a good friend (the matron of honour, perhaps) should be up to date with the situation and should be the point of contact for guests, should any last minute emergencies occur.

When you (and where appropriate, your parents) have made your list, you can then choose the venue that will accommodate the number of guests you want. At this point you'll probably need to cut the list. Do you *really* want that old school friend you haven't seen for fifteen years? Or the work-mate whom you just know is a nasty gossipmonger? Or your father's football or golf buddies? A good yardstick to measure this by is that your parents' friends and family should be people well known to at least one, if not both of you. That should cut down on any unnecessary guests. This is the time to be ruthless. Of course there are a lot of familial obligations, but this is *your* day and you should have people you love, or at least like, sharing it with you.

Bearing in mind you'll probably go well over it, you *must* try and set a realistic budget. Weddings can cost very little (just the price of the licence and registrar, two friends as witnesses, then drinks and sandwiches in a pub) or they can be astronomically expensive. Two weeks after our own wedding, Percy and I went to Liza Minelli and David Gest's wedding in New York. It was lavish indeed and there was great attention to detail, too. In contrast with ours, it was held in a church, with 1,200 guests. The reception was in another venue an hour away, requiring transportation, and the 25 bridesmaids and groomsmen and various other guests had to be flown over from different parts of the world. In comparison, ours was a small family affair!

Usually, the bride's family pays for the wedding, the reception, the transportation, the flowers, the music, the stationery and the wedding dress. The groom pays for the rings, the gifts for the wedding party (matron of honour, best man, bridesmaids, groomsmen, parents, etc.), the flowers for the bride and her attendants, and the honeymoon. Or, if there are no parents involved, you can pay for the wedding equally.

WHAT TO BUDGET FOR

It's essential to list absolutely *everything* you will be paying for and to obtain at least two written estimates. Here is my checklist.

Church or Registry Office.

Wedding venue for reception, lunch or dinner.

Wedding dress and accessories.

Flowers.

Transportation.

Food and drink (and this will *invariably* go over budget – ours certainly did).

Disc jockey or band (or both).

Rings.

Photographer and video.

Invitations and printing (placecards, menus, etc.).

Bridesmaids' dresses, hired suits for the groom and best man.

Gifts/party favours.

The honeymoon.

There are bound to be more hidden costs so you will definitely need several quotations for each item. When the smelling salts have revived you from the total cost of all this, you could consider some money-saving ideas:

Instead of a photographer or videographer, have a friend take pictures. (Make sure they don't drink!)

Cut the guest list – I know it's hard, but you have to.

Change the venue. If you're really strapped for cash, instead of a hotel (they are *so* expensive, especially where the food and drink is concerned), have the reception in someone's garden.

Instead of a sit-down dinner, have finger food that an aunt or a friend will help prepare. Here are some favourites:

• Sausages on sticks
• Quail's eggs (not as expensive as you might think)
• Mini pizzas (you can buy them at the supermarket)
• Asparagus spears with vinaigrette dip
• Smoked salmon on toast triangles
• Cheese straws (you can get really fancy ones)
• Crudités with a dip (although this can be messy).

Instead of champagne, just serve wine or beer, or sparkling wine. (Many people don't care for champagne anyway – myself among them. If they're having fun they won't miss it.)

Ask a teenage brother or sister, cousin or a young friend who might be inclined to be DJ for the night. He (or she) will relish the opportunity to be the coolest guy (or chick) at the reception. But *do* tell him (or her) exactly what to play and discuss it at length in advance. We actually drew up a play list of seventies and eighties

Disco with our DJ, which was excellently supplemented by his own choices. It's incredible how popular eighties Disco is across all generations because it's lively, fresh and upbeat. The moment Gloria Gaynor started wailing 'I Will Survive', our dance floor was packed. Some other particular Disco favourites we played were Abba's 'Dancing Queen' (and other Abba hits), everything from the Bee Gees' 'Saturday Night Fever' to Streisand and Donna Summer's 'Enough is Enough' and Aretha Franklin's 'Respect'.

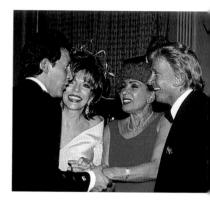

Greeting some of our wedding guests. The author, Dame Shirley Bassey and friend, trying to hold the groom steady.

Instead of flowers, decorate the room with balloons and streamers. It can look very pretty and there are a variety of paper tablecloths and napkins available from stationery shops.

Make your own wedding dress (or have a local dressmaker do it). You can buy fabulous patterns to copy, often by the top designers, and at your nearest fabric shop there will be a list of dressmakers who specialise in bridal gowns. Again, don't forget to get an estimate first. Or try one of the many places where you can hire wedding gowns and accessories. As for the ring, instead of buying it at an expensive jeweller, visit one of the flea markets or local markets such as Portobello Road or Camden Passage in London, and any of the downtown open-air markets in New York, and the car boot (garage) sales held all over America. There are always a few stalls selling vintage rings, which are often far more attractive than modern versions and these can mean a big saving.

Instead of sending printed invitations prepare a well designed fax giving all the details and send that to everyone you have invited. Most people have access to faxes and if they don't have one, then use the telephone. It may not be the last word in etiquette, but it's cost-friendly!

Our wedding went off without a hitch because we'd planned it so meticulously and we also gave ourselves enough time on the day of the wedding to deal with any last minute emergencies. Six weeks before the event I started arranging the table placements in my head, even though I wasn't sure yet whether everyone we had invited would be able to attend. Then, into a four-hole binder, I wrote out the complete guest list on page one and then put ten to twelve numbered names on separate pages, making sure the people I was seating together would be compatible with each other. Do this with your fiancé – it may well be your first fight, but placement is *crucial* and I think one of the successes of our wedding was that dozens of people told us, 'Oh, I was at the *best* table. It was so much fun.' The fact was everyone had fun, most of all Percy and I.

We planned our colour scheme in great detail. I chose to wear a lilac silk dress, which I designed myself with *Dynasty* dress designer Nolan Miller and Mark Zunnino. I wanted the colours and flowers in the dining room to complement the dress. We decided to have purple velvet tablecloths and silver bamboo chairs with lilac seat covers. The white napkins were tied with lavender ribbon and the menus were on deep lilac paper printed in silver ink, while the place cards were also purple and slotted into tiny silver frames, which everyone was given as a keepsake.

I love flowers and if you can afford to be extravagant, they can really make the room look fantastic. The flowers for our wedding cost an absolute fortune, but they were worth it. In the middle of each table were tall vases filled with lilac-coloured water and in them stood masses of Casablanca lilies, white orchids and trailing jasmine. Green grapes were scattered on the tablecloth at the foot of the vases, as were a dozen tiny tea-lights. The room in which we were married was lit by candlelight. As it was February, it was dark by the five o'clock ceremony so the room looked glowing and beautiful. There were huge swathes of lilies and white lilac everywhere, on the mirrors and in

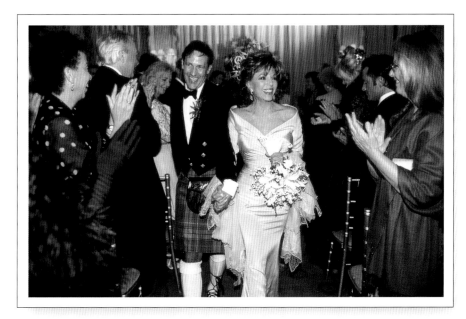

Here comes the bride –
and we all couldn't be
happier.

Below left: One of the
tables at Claridge's
with its flower name.

Below right: This
gorgeous wedding cake
tasted as good as it
looked.

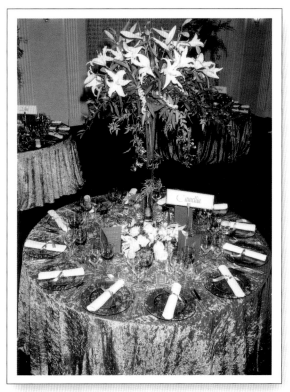

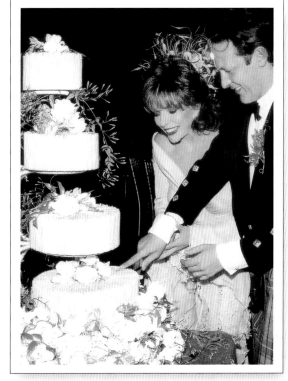

enormous vases each side of the altar, and on the backs of chairs and lining the aisle. The guests all sat on silver chairs, which were later moved into the dining room.

I disliked the idea of the tables being numbered (those on Number One will think theirs is the best while those on Number Fifteen think they're in social Siberia). Instead, we decided to give our tables flower names: Lily of the Valley, Gardenia, Poppy, Orchid, etc. This was quite original and everyone seemed happy with where they sat.

I gave much thought to my bridal bouquet. After telling our excellent florist, Steel Magnolias, what I liked, they sent over two different options to try out the week before, along with two examples for table centrepieces. This way, I was able to sit with the florist to add and subtract flowers to get the exact effect I wanted for the bouquet and the tables. Most good florists will do this for you at a small extra cost and it's well worth it.

My bouquet was exquisite, consisting of lily of the valley (my favourite flower), white lilies, freesias and a little bit of pale lilac. Around the base was wrapped an antique white lace handkerchief, given to me by a dear friend, which was my 'something old'.

On our wedding day over 3,000 blooms filled Claridge's reception rooms and, as Nolan Miller (who had flown in from LA) remarked, 'There can't be a single lily or orchid left in Europe!' Throughout the night the subtle scent of flowers filled the air and when I entered the room where we were to be married, I was stunned by their gorgeous effect.

We were delighted after the wedding that we had decided to have everything videotaped. We particularly wanted the video cameraman to shoot our guests arriving at Claridge's and at the reception when Percy and I were having our pictures taken. Later, we were able to watch so many conversations and things we had missed at the time. The cameraman also filmed Percy getting ready with his best man, Chris Pennington, and myself with my matron of honour, Judy Bryer, my daughters Tara and Katy, my hairdresser, couturiers and various girl friends in my hotel room preparing for the ceremony.

Because I wanted to oversee every single detail I stayed at Claridge's the night before so that when the flowers and the table arrangements arrived in the early morning I would be there to supervise. Also, since I had agonised over my table placements so much, I wanted to personally place the tiny frames.

One of the most important aspects of a wedding is the music and Percy and I had spent a great deal of time choosing it. Actually, every single thing is important but we wanted particular music throughout. Because Percy is half-Scottish and he and most male members of his family would be wearing kilts, we thought a touch of the bagpipes would be appropriate, so we had Jim Motherwell, the Queen's personal piper, play during the evening.

As the guests arrived and were seated, and up until the moment I arrived, we had our DJ play nostalgic forties classics such as Frank Sinatra and our favourite Steve Tyrell songs, 'Give Me the Simple Life', 'On the Sunny Side of the Street', 'The Very Thought of You', 'I Can't Give You Anything But Love, Baby' and 'I've Got the World on a String'. Mellow and romantic, it suited the environment. Then, as I entered with Max Bryer, who was giving me away, and his wife, Judy, the DJ played the 'Triumphal March and Ballet Music' from Verdi's Aida, which was extremely stirring. During the signing of the register he played Handel's 'The Arrival of the Queen of Sheba' and when the ceremony was over Mendelssohn's classic 'Wedding March' as we walked ecstatically down the aisle as man and wife. There are so many choices of wedding music, but you and your fiancé must spend the time choosing what works for you – I assure you it's well worth it.

Our registrar, Alison Cathcart, gave us several choices for our wedding vows, which we mixed and matched and added some of our own words so it was tailored especially for us.

Try to get a professional photograph of all your guests, or at least as many as possible. During the cocktail reception a photographer was busy shooting everyone in that room while the superb and rapid-fire Brian Aris, specially commissioned by *OK!* Magazine to cover the wedding, shot us in another. A few weeks later we were able to give each guest (those who weren't camera shy) a memento of our fantastic day, which they all appreciated.

Shortly after the reception with a flourish of bagpipes Mr and Mrs Gibson were then ushered into the dining room, which looked absolutely exquisite. The fourteen tables were set up around the dance floor, in the middle of which stood the cake. Aah, the cake! Isn't that delicious treat synonymous with weddings? Again, the choice was endless. Siobhan, our wedding planner, had shown us brochures and asked us what we wanted taste-wise and frenzied discussions ensued. The cake we finally chose was a gorgeous four-tiered confection made of white chocolate curls enveloping a luscious dark chocolate Suchard filling. It was trimmed with white roses, jasmine and pale lilac freesias. When we had our first dance to our favourite song, 'The Way You Look Tonight', an emotional sigh surged from the guests and before we knew it the floor was filled with our friends, who were all eager to dance the night away.

OUR WEDDING MENU

The food at our reception was superb. Three weeks previously (the day after our engagement party and we were *extremely* hung over) we chose and discussed the menu at Claridge's. The chef called this little ceremony 'a tasting'. That way, we knew *exactly* what we were going to get and how delicious it was. Here's what we had:

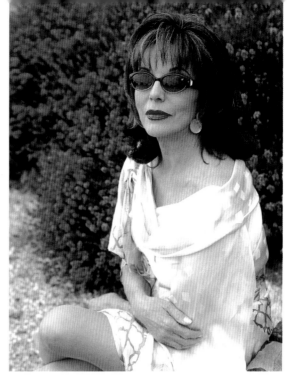

Right: Looking forward to another party. (Grayshott Hall, 2002).

Below: The good life of St Tropez. Paul, the patron, pours the champagne for Charles Delevingne and the author hosting a launch party at Le Voile Rouge (St Tropez, 1998).

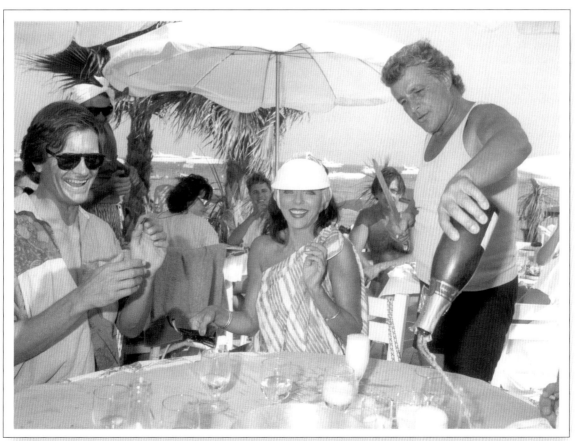

- Ballotine of Foie Gras with Pistachios, Salad of French Beans with Mâche (known as Lamb's Lettuce here) and Vinaigrette. Brioche.
- Vegetarian alternative: Crown of Asparagus with Avocado and Sweet Pepper Oil.
- Noisettes of Lamb with Glazed Artichokes, Morels and Port Mustard, Baby Broccoli and Gratin of Swedes and Potatoes.
- Vegetarian alternative: Baked Artichoke with Wild Mushroom Ragoût under a Golden Dome of Puff Pastry.
- Assiettes of Desserts.

Then came the speeches, probably the most emotional and joyous part of a wedding after the ceremony. The father of the bride, (or whomever gives the bride away), makes the first speech, and Max's was touching. Percy's speech brought tears to everyone's eyes, especially mine – it was so wonderfully moving. After that, Chris, our best man, spoke with wit and charm, and finally, I wanted to say a few words, although it isn't usual for the bride to speak (well, you know me!).

The dancing continued until the wee hours. Our guests were a mixture of all ages from eight to 80, but absolutely everyone was hot to trot. In fact, we didn't stop dancing all night. The Kevin Baker Orchestra interspersed their jazzy Sinatra and show tunes with the DJ's Disco sounds and we were even lucky enough to have Shirley Bassey sing a *cappella*, a brilliant version of 'And I Love You So'. We danced everything from the Gay Gordons to the conga, and I can truthfully say I have never had a more wonderful and memorable day. May yours be as good. However, one word of warning: we *did* go over budget by 20 per cent but apparently this is perfectly normal – so watch everything!

CHILDREN'S BIRTHDAY PARTIES

As a parent, I know that organising a child's party can be very rewarding, but extremely exhausting. The inevitable chaos they leave behind is a small price to pay for sharing their excitement. There are four golden rules for giving a good children's party, be it for three-year-olds or thirteen-year-olds:

Keep it short (no more than two and a half hours).

Keep it sweet (give them lots of goodies to eat and to hell with the dentist, at least for a day).

Keep it small (no more than fifteen or you'll go crazy).

And keep them smiling (or so busy they don't have time to cry).

If possible, it's fun to have the party outside, and they should be at teatime. I always had my own children's birthday parties start at 2.30 p.m. and finish promptly at 5 p.m. Unlike adults, children usually arrive on time so we'd start a series of games as soon as possible. For three- to eight-year-olds Grandmother's Footsteps or musical chairs are oldies but goodies, and all kids love them. Forty minutes of that and then it would be teatime, for which the table would always be set with the appropriate age-related, or icon-of-the-week theme – Mickey Mouse, Batman, Barbie Doll, *Jungle Book* and Action Man were all themes I used for Tara, Katy and Sacha. Today, for the girls it would probably be a Britney Spears dress-up competition and for the boys some sort of *Star Wars* or technology theme.

Tea would consist of little triangular-shaped sandwiches of either scrambled egg, tuna fish, smoked salmon or grated cheese with the crusts cut off, cookies, jam tarts and chocolate fingers and individual containers of jelly plus lots of Smarties scattered on the table then, of course, the *pièce de résistance*, the birthday cake arriving complete with blazing candles.

There would be balloons galore and little toys and novelties for the guests and immediately after tea the entertainer would arrive. There were no videos when my kids were small so they were content to watch conjurers, Punch and Judy shows, magicians or clowns.

Today the average five-year-old is quite sophisticated. Although they may be ready to see an Ali G or Michael Jackson impersonator or have a hair-braiding expert teach them the tricks of the trade, a Tweenie or Barney party with face-painting competitions or a *Toy Story* costume contest (Who's the Best Buzz Lightyear?) is more appropriate and should be quite popular with small kids. You can easily buy the cakes, theme plates and decorations from any supermarket, and the choice is endless.

With only 30 minutes to go, you're probably tearing your hair out as the little darlings get rowdier and temper tantrums abound. It's amazing how temperamental four-year-olds can become, so it's *essential* to have a lot of help on the day. I reckon a ratio of one adult per three kids is about right, and you'll still need a stiff drink at the end of the day when you collapse.

The last half hour of my parties we used to play either Musical Chairs, Hide and Seek (don't forget to hide the breakable ornaments!) or Pass the Parcel, but today's kids will probably want to watch a video. Try the games, though. It's more rewarding although more exhausting to watch them frolic about instead of slumping in front of the television set.

Thank God for the doorbell when the first of the mothers, carers or nannies arrives for prompt pick-up. Give each child a present, usually a bag with several appropriate little toys and one or two sweets (candies) in it, then it's goodbye until the next child's birthday (which in my case was only six weeks later). Help!

Since my children are now past the age of kids' parties, I've been giving an annual children's Christmas party for some of my friends' children, my eight godchildren and my little granddaughter, Miel, who is now old enough to be included. It's usually just tea and juice, a vast amount of cakes and cookies, and helping me to decorate the tree. The guests range from two years old to fourteen. Sometimes I'll have a male friend dress up as Santa and come in with a sack of presents but it's all convivial and jolly, and the kids like catching up with one another, as do the parents and they all get a present from under the tree at the end.

COCKTAIL PARTIES

The secret to a great drinks party is to invite masses of people, more than you need in fact, and to make absolutely make sure that you have enough waiters or helpers so that your guests' glasses are never empty. The best time to hold a drinks party is between 6.30 and 9 p.m. Most people will stay about an hour so it will be staggered anyway (or else they'll be the ones staggering).

It's usual to serve hors d'oeuvres (or dead-bits-on-toast, as I call them) during a drinks party. These should be small enough to be eaten in one bite, not gloopy or covered in sauce. Make sure you have a ton of them. As a guest there's nothing more annoying than to see the last tiny potato stuffed with caviar disappear into someone else's mouth, or even worse to watch in vain that last sausage being gobbled up.

It's much easier to serve just wine and soft drinks because if you start getting into 'real' cocktails such as Manhattans, Martinis or even simple G and T's you'd better have several barmen, more skilled than Tom Cruise in *Cocktail*, available.

Music isn't necessary at a drinks party. In fact, it's a distraction – the conversations alone should be music to everyone's ears. You can mix up people of all ages and professions as much as you like and it's a good time to rid yourself of any social obligations. Make sure the room isn't too hot and that you've left enough ashtrays around. Even if you disapprove, there are still a lot of smokers out there, particularly when drinking.

Unless you want squiffy guests to linger past their sell-by date, stop serving drinks fifteen or twenty minutes after the given hour. Last of all: don't worry. If you've made sure you have enough drink and canapés, and that your staff or servers are skilled, relax and enjoy the show.

DINNER PARTIES

I've found it almost impossible to give a civilised sit-down dinner in Hollywood. In a town notorious for its bad social manners, there are always no-shows, but in Britain it's much easier as people *do* understand that cancelling at the eleventh hour is terribly rude, not to mention a nightmare for the hostess.

I give several types of dinner parties. Once a year I throw a Christmas party in which I serve a buffet (because of the size of my flat I can only invite 50 or 60 guests). I want everyone to be able to sit down reasonably comfortably, even if they have to balance plates on their laps. I invite my closest friends and sometimes, new people – friends don't necessarily want to see the same old faces every year. I'm quite ruthless over whom I choose to invite, too. Bores are definitely out, as are obligatory business people (with them I'll have lunch at a restaurant).

I make sure I have the most delicious food possible and I am lucky enough to have a marvellous chef, who will come in and cook memorable food. As it's a buffet I like to have at least eight or nine different dishes on the menu so that everyone has a choice. Some ideas for menus are:

A Christmas theme for one of the author's buffets.

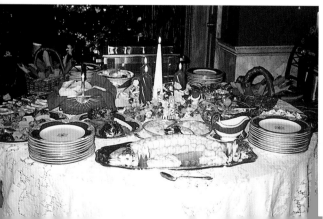

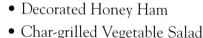

- Decorated Honey Ham
- Char-grilled Vegetable Salad
- Tzatsiki Salad
- Salmon en Croûte
- Beef Stroganoff
- Chicken with Mango and Mint Dressing served with brown rice or Chicken Cacciatore

- Pecan Pie with Rocky Road Ice Cream
- Chocolate Roulade
- Crème Brûlée
- Sherry Trifle
- Chocolate and Raspberry Tart

These are all heaven, but a calorific nightmare but at Christmas I throw caution to the winds and the puddings are so scrumptious that everyone has at least three portions, so beware! I also bring in several excellently trained bartenders, who have strict instructions not let anyone's glass stay empty.

Some of my Christmas ornaments are over 30 years old, but I also buy new ones each year.

The dining room is also where my tall Christmas tree stands, heavily decorated by my family and me, and loaded with all of the baubles and ornaments I've been collecting and making ever since my children were little.

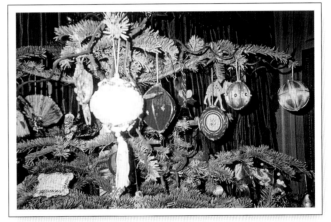

For my Christmas soirée I encourage women to dress glamorously since I love getting dressed up. Anyway, at Christmas time I feel it's particularly appropriate. It's an effort to give a really great party so why not encourage everyone to look gorgeous in celebration of the festivities? Plus the men like it, too!

My apartment is always decorated to the hilt with flowers and plants such as white poinsettias, azaleas and jasmine, and I'll also have Christmas decorations and candles. I try to get rid of as much clutter as I can, so some of my bulkier ornaments get shoved in the closet and the furniture is moved around for maximum space.

Most people at my Christmas party know each other so the atmosphere is convivial, and crowded. Invited for 8 p.m., I try to have the buffet on the table by 9.15, although some guests can be

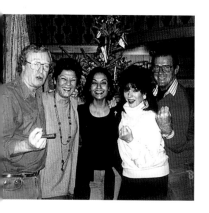

Michael Caine, Jan Gold, Shakira Caine, yours truly and Roger Moore ready to punch the photographer (Christmas, 1999).

notoriously tardy. However, I don't believe in waiting for latecomers because that's unfair to those guests who *were* punctual and who are starving by 9.30.

I even have a couple of tables set up in my bedroom so that there are plenty of places to sit. Usually everyone has a wonderful time and the party goes on and on. For the past two years I hired a South American band who played Sambas, Salsas, Tangos and Cha-Chas. They were terrific, if a tiny bit too loud. Unfortunately, one year a neighbour called the police at 1 a.m., so the band had to stop playing earlier than we wanted. Maybe I'll try line-dancing next year?

SIT-DOWN DINNERS

Whenever I give an interview in which I mention my cooking, people look amazed. Contrary to public opinion, I'm quite a nifty cook and there are three or four simple dishes I specialise in. Since Percy and I married we share the cooking chores, particularly my world-famous spaghetti bolognaise. So here it is folks – and if you're slimming, eat a mini-portion:

Heat 50g (2oz, ¼ cup) butter, 1 tablespoon olive oil and 1 large chopped onion in a large saucepan. Then brown 225g (8oz, 1 cup) each of ground chuck beef, ground pork and ground veal. Add half a green pepper (deseeded and chopped), 4 cloves of crushed mint garlic, 2 cans of tomato paste, 1 400g (14oz) can of chopped tomatoes (best bought from an Italian store, ditto the spaghetti), ½ tablespoon Worcestershire sauce, a pinch of sugar, 125ml (4fl oz, ½ cup) of Chianti and salt and pepper to taste. Cover this brew and cook very slowly over a low heat, stirring regularly, for at least 3 hours. Make the spaghetti according to the directions on the package and serve up! They'll come back for second helpings for sure.

We also love a chicken dish that is *really* simple to do. It's healthy, and great for Sunday lunch. The size of the chicken will depend on how many guests you're having and will determine how long you cook it. Here it is:

First, preheat the oven to 225°C (425°F/gas mark 7). Stuff your chicken with sausage meat or sage stuffing from your butcher. Some supermarkets make a pretty good chicken that is already pre-stuffed. Place it in a baking pan, along with enough new potatoes and onions for everyone. I particularly like smaller onions (allow one per person) that can be put in whole, otherwise just quarter up some large ones. Rub the chicken, as well as dousing the potatoes and onions with masses of virgin olive oil, then sprinkle a tiny amount of salt and (if you want to) pepper over everything. Place in the oven.

Now here's where my husband and I diverge. I like to baste the chicken every half hour (I usually buy a chicken that takes ½ to 1¼ hours to roast), and he likes to leave it pretty much alone to baste in its own juices, maybe basting it twice after the first hour. Experiment to see what you like best. Then just cook up some greens (peas, Brussels sprouts or broccoli). Make the gravy from the olive oil left in the pan and gravy powder by placing a saucepan over low heat, covering about 2.5cm (1in) with an equal mixture of the pan juices and water. Add the powder and stir vigorously. It's easy.

Calves liver Italian-style is also excellent. If you're feeling daring, add a couple of slices of fried bacon (very naughty, but very nice, occasionally).

Mix 3 tablespoons flour with a dash of pepper and a pinch of salt. Dredge the liver in this mixture and then lightly sauté with a few sliced onions in olive oil until it's slightly pink. Take it off the heat and add 1 tablespoon margarine, 3 tablespoons lemon juice and ½ teaspoon grated rind (apparently some thyme disguises the liver flavour, but I happen to like it) to the pan, which should have all the juices still in it. Pour the sauce over the liver and serve with mixed vegetables and mashed potatoes.

Kitchen suppers are great fun. Although I call it a 'Kitchen Supper', my kitchen isn't big enough for everyone to sit down, so we serve ourselves straight from the kitchen and then take it to the dining room table. We usually invite no more than eight or ten guests (only family or extremely close friends) and we do everything ourselves, even the washing up (well, we *do* have a dishwasher!).

FORMAL SIT-DOWN DINNERS

I've rather gone off the idea of giving formal sit-down dinners. It's an awful lot of effort and organisation when frankly it's easier to take guests out to The Ivy when we're in London or Spago in LA. However, when I do give dinners, I discuss the menu with the chef two or three weeks in advance. I make sure that the wines are excellent, too, and that I have masses of flowers and candles around. Then I cross my fingers and hope on the night that no one will cancel or be horribly late. I have found that in the past twenty years or so people seem much more cavalier about cancelling or turning up late, which may be part of my disappointment with formal sit-downs. It's rather sad, really, because a good dinner party, with the intimacy one never gets in a restaurant, stimulating guests and varied conversation, can be truly exhilarating.

And my final word on entertainment comes from my friend Sue Mengers, who applies the 'if they don't invite you after you've invited them, don't ask them back again' principle, a school of thought which I wholly embrace. However, there are certain allowances I make for friends who perhaps can't afford to entertain, but at least make the effort to telephone and check in regularly.

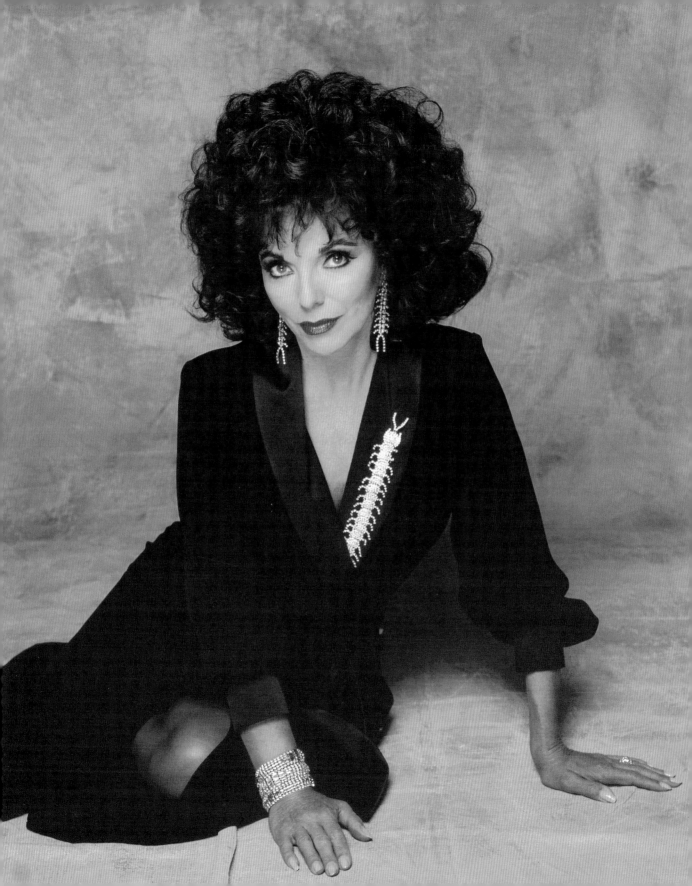

The pursuit of happiness

Happiness is everyone's ultimate goal, but what is this elusive thing for which we all search? Some might say it's the absence of pain, so if you have experienced physical or mental pain in your life, getting rid of it should definitely make you happier. Many studies have shown that the happiest people are those who live for the moment, and who celebrate *every* moment of their life. Unhappy people *think* they could find happiness if they had great riches or great beauty, but certainly some of the richest and most beautiful people in the world have lived terribly unhappy lives. But in the long term the happiness we strive for should not be so hard to achieve. Happiness is not a given: we can appreciate it more if we don't have it all the time. And I don't think we're meant to have it all the time because life is a mixture of highs and lows, and only when you've experienced the lows can you appreciate the highs.

I actually believe that people were happier years ago when there were not so many activities to choose from. People are encouraged to do so much, what with concerts, television, movies, shopping (seven days a week), football, pubs, magazines (there are hundreds of them) and newspapers (with ten national papers, Britain has the most newspapers in the world). There's so much to do and so little time to do it in.

There is a Scottish proverb that goes, 'Be happy while you're living, for you're a long time dead.' But that's the trouble: time. No one seems to have enough time to do all the things they'd like to do today. So many people seem to be wandering around on remote control, yet they can't find the remote. But some people *are* living life to the full and are truly happy. Their happiness doesn't depend on a mantelpiece clogged with 'stiffies' and a full date book of exciting trips, and fine restaurants to go to. *Whatever age you are and whatever your means*, real happiness comes from being satisfied with your own personal growth and trying to achieve your long-term goals. And those goals can be as ambitious or as minor as you choose. Don't let others tell you what to do to make yourself happy. If you weigh 200 pounds, are happy about it and not in bad health, don't allow anyone else to con you into trying to be a size eight. If it isn't *your own* motivation that spurs you into making changes, it's not going to make you any happier to make them because others think you should.

One of the things to face in life is that you cannot control everything that happens. And there are some things you can *never* change. You can't alter your height or the colour of your skin but there are many things you *can* alter. Make a list of what you want to achieve, even if it's as simple as losing five pounds or learning to swim, because small achievements spur you on to bigger ones. For example, when I started writing short stories and essays at school I never believed I would have the patience to finish anything. I found the thought of writing an entire book incredibly daunting until I wrote my first, *Past Imperfect*, in 1978. Well, I buckled down, believing in my ability (even if some others didn't) and I finished my autobiography. It became a bestseller (hurrah!), and since then I've written ten more books. Of course there's enormous discipline and hard work involved, but absolutely *nothing* comes easy in this life and everything that is worth having is *worth* working hard towards.

Often you may feel out of control because you can't stop worrying. Anxiety haunts you and fills your dreams with angst. But you must realise that *all* creatures worry. Animals in the jungle probably worry more than any other mammal. Think about it – any minute they could be someone's lunch! Many things happen in life that we don't want to happen but you have to learn to deal with them. In fact, as a human being you are actually programmed to deal with stress, death, problems and anxiety to a greater extent than you might think.

Man (and woman) is a tough and hardy creature who, throughout the ages, has become soft. Mankind either invented, discovered, or found a way to exploit (for better or worse) practically everything on this planet, yet most people today are unable to even fix a fence, let alone any part of their dwelling that's in disrepair. Yes, we drive cars and work computers, and make complicated travel arrangements but what our ancestors accomplished were *major achievements*: discovering fire (yes!), inventing the wheel, and domesticating animals for labour, farming and every kind of tool from weapons to hammers, building all sorts of abodes from mud huts to castles. Mankind did all this and *taught* himself to do it, too. They were the most astounding accomplishments. But today, with obvious exceptions, the average man is no longer creative. So many things have been invented already and often he can't even change a tyre, a fuse, or paint a room.

KEEP IT IN PERSPECTIVE

When I feel down and depressed (which is rare) I make myself focus on the tragedies and meaningless loss of life happening in the world today. It doesn't take long for me to get back on track and realise just how lucky I am and how happy I am because of it. To love and be loved is the greatest happiness of all and one of the things in life that makes me the happiest is to be in a loving relationship. The intimacy that comes with this does give great cause for happiness.

Friends are another reason to be happy. Maybe you think you don't have enough. Make some more – start with your neighbours, they may be on a similar wavelength to you as you live in the same area. Don't be shy, make the effort. It could be worth it and you'll never know if you don't try.

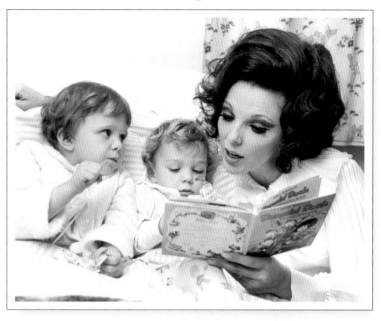

Try not to fight with your loved ones or family – or anyone else for that matter. I *hate* conflict (contrary to the popular misconception of Alexis). Road rage, air rage and all the rages we're prone to are useless expenditures of valuable energy that we could put towards becoming a happier individual. Sometimes, however, it is healthy to blow off steam rather than let things simmer, so use your judgement about this.

A simple pleasure used to be reading my toddlers bedtime stories before I went out on the town.

Unfortunately, we know that there are people out there who actively seek out conflicts and almost enjoy them. In our crime-ridden society conflicts are endemic and all too horrible. Since angry people are usually frightened people, they often take out their fears in anger towards others. For example, the Cowardly Lion in *The Wizard of Oz* was scary until Dorothy said 'Boo' to him, then he crumbled and became a jelly. If you stand up to people, particularly bullies, they, too, will often crumble. Unhappy people are often

212 | JOAN'S WAY

bullies and sadists because their goal is to make other people as unhappy as they are. Don't let them do that to you: you are the mistress of your destiny – *you* have the power to be happy so keep those people out of your life. As Joseph Conrad said, 'You shall judge a man by his foes as well as by his friends'. A happy person doesn't want conflict, doesn't need it.

Be open to change. It's the only constant in life. Everything in the world changes radically. Go with the flow, accept changes but be your own person in spite of them.

MY TIPS FOR HAPPINESS

Here are some of my guidelines that can make you happy.

Make time for fun – a game of cards, darts or Scrabble, a night out at the movies or a concert. Be the instigator, you don't have to wait to be asked.

Spend an evening alone, just pampering yourself – a warm scented bath surrounded by candles and a cool jazz CD, or classical music playing. Then put on your favourite video, *Gone with the Wind* or *Some Like it Hot*, and sip a delicious glass of wine – very happy-making.

Don't agonise over past failures, and don't cry over spilt milk. What's done is done. As Scarlett O'Hara says, 'I'll think about that tomorrow; tomorrow is another day.' Onward!

Keep trying to reach your goals and potential. Don't *ever* give up – *ever*. Make plans even if they might be a touch unrealistic. One of the keys to being happy is to believe in a beautiful future. Hope springs eternal.

Spend time with your family. It can be extremely rewarding. Seek out a cousin or an aunt you haven't seen for years. Maybe you'll find a new friend there.

Live life to the fullest and appreciate what you have. Make a list of the good things in your life – it could be longer than you think.

Some people think if they had a better job, they would be happy. If you're dissatisfied with your job, find one you like. Get connected to one that suits your interests and become involved in it. The more involved and interested you are in what you're doing, the more chance you have of rising or getting a promotion.

Love yourself with all your faults. As Max Ehrmann wrote in the inspirational *Desiderata*, 'You are a child of the universe, no less than the trees and the stars, you have a right to be here. With all its sham, drudgery and broken dreams it is still a beautiful world. Strive to be happy.'

And finally, stop moaning. Choose to be happy and take responsibility for the choices *you* make in life.

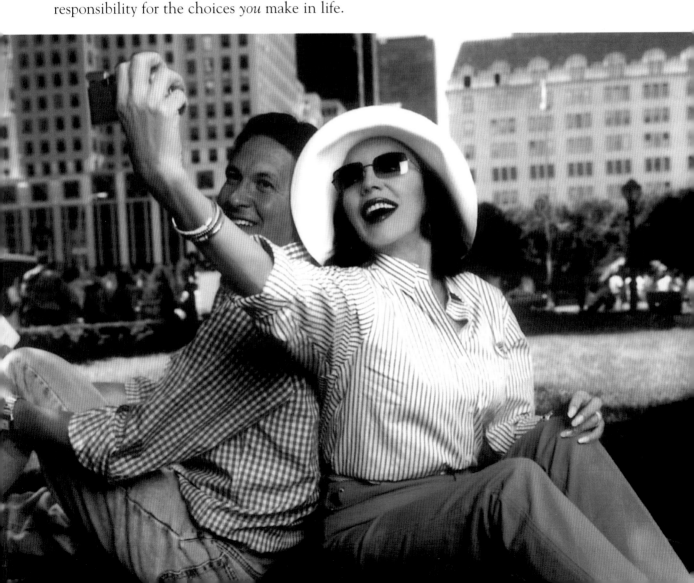

Taking a bite out of the Big Apple – the author and her soon-to-be husband in Central Park, New York, 2001.

With age comes wisdom

(or the advantages of getting older)

There are so many positive things that come from getting older: certainly wisdom, knowledge and tolerance, and the older I get the more I realise how little I know, when in the arrogance of my youth I thought I knew a lot. I'm amazed today at so many young people who think they know it all, when really all they know is who was *Top of the Pops* last week and what Britney Spears or David Beckham's latest hairstyle is.

There are many virtues that the young *do* possess, but wisdom is usually not one of them. After all, how can you be truly wise, if you haven't lived long enough to gain experience?

Hopefully as we grow older, tolerance is one of the things we learn. I know I've always been a touch on the impatient side (a touch!). It's genetic, inherited from my father and being a volatile Gemini contributes to this. I remember at age five or six walking down a crowded street with my mother and becoming really cross at being bumped into by people. Now of course I just try to dodge them.

I have noticed a tremendous intolerance today towards others, sadly, often from young people. My driver, Steve Drake, who's been with me for years, is incredibly tolerant towards other drivers, who often cut in front of him, give him 'the finger' or verbal abuse, just because he's an excellent driver who obeys the rules of the road to the letter. Interesting that most road accidents are usually caused by young people, particularly aggressive young men. As you get older you realise how stupid other drivers can be and how precious life is, so you don't take so many risks.

Babies aren't born with compassion towards others. They are born behaving like little animals wanting to be fed and watered whenever they want and yelling until they get it. Children need discipline – it's essential.

Reading about the young Royal Princesses Elizabeth and Margaret, growing up in the thirties and forties, I was amazed at how strictly they were brought up and how few treats they had. They didn't go on summer holidays and were only allowed to see one pantomime a year. Instead, the Princesses relied on their imagination to amuse themselves, as did most children of that generation. A child today would go on strike if that was his or her life. Even the poorest of children have a TV and video machine and several toys, if not a computer, and holidays are taken for granted. Children today rule the roost and they know it, too. Advertisements, commercials and many commodities are geared towards them, as are television series and mainstream movies, in which more often than not a moppet plays an important role. Watch television early in the morning and practically every channel will be showing cartoons, interspersed with merchandise aimed at seducing two- to twelve-year-olds into persuading their parents to buy them. And it works.

Children choose their meals now and even what goes in the refrigerator. It's an exceptional child that sits at the table, finishing everything on its plate without watching the box at the same time. Some supermarkets even have miniature wheel baskets so that the little darlings can choose their own chow and fill it up with goodies (usually junk food) right next to Mama's.

It's sad but true that in some parts of the Western world we have a new breed of youngsters with little or no respect for authority, discipline or their elders. Youth crime is soaring while in Britain the 'yobbo' generation of the late teens and twenty-somethings has made it the weekend fashion to drink until they're sick (usually on someone else's property), to urinate in the streets and even make love in public.

This does not seem to hold true in France, Italy and Spain, where children still have respect for their families and aren't allowed to do whatever they want, wherever they want. And in the States young children seem better behaved. It seems hard to believe that Britain was once the world's model for dignity, manners, etiquette and civil behaviour. What happened? It's tragic to think that discipline and respect went by the board.

I honestly believe that discipline is the key to raising a happy, well-adjusted child who has respect for others. You have to be cruel sometimes to be kind, as my parents used to tell me as they stopped me stuffing sweets (candies) in my mouth before lunch.

It was gratifying to see the respect that was given to the Queen Mother at her funeral, so perhaps there's hope for us yet, but the rudeness and change in attitude today is alarming. Change was anathema to the Queen Mother. I realise that change is essential, however, it seems to me that everything we have held dear in England is being ditched in favour of what the young want: being trendy, breaking rules, not conforming to the values and standards that have made civilised society and without the clear, well stated purpose of

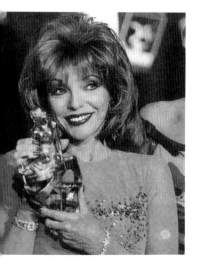

Receiving la Nymphe d'Honneur at the Monte Carlo Television Festival. (Monaco, 2001)

the youth of other decades. Basically, cocking a snook for the sake of it at authority, whether it's the police, the schools or anyone who tells them there's perhaps a better way. This seemed particularly apparent to me at the more recent May Day celebrations, where such disparate protest groups congregate to further their own very specific and no doubt worthy cause. 'We protest at globalisation because… it's a danger to the whales… No, wait, to the rainforest… No, wait, to labour unions in developed countries… No, wait, to the poor and marginalised in underdeveloped countries… No, wait…' There's serious need for a consensus here!

For example, as a child I went to football games with my father. I thought they were extremely boring, but the players did seem to treat each other with courtesy and a sense of fair play. Today, football pitches look like a war zone and it seems the norm for the players to attack each other viciously. As for football hooligans, are they human, or have they descended from another planet?

There is only one you. Even though over 6 billion people inhabit our world, there is still no one at all who is any way like you. You are unique and you should realise that. Some people may look alike, but no two people are ever *exactly* alike.

The French novelist Colette said, 'What a wonderful life I've had. I only wish I'd realised it sooner!' And life *is* wonderful, even with all the suffering, horror and tragedy that goes on in the world. It's sad that so many people only look on the dark side and of course it's so easy to do. When you wake in the morning and see the cluttered bedside table and old newspapers on the carpet, which needs vacuuming, and your clothes strewn all over the place, you see the worst and probably want to pull the bedcovers over you and go back to sleep. But if you look on the bright side the scenario can change. Feel how comfortable your bed is, isn't that the sun shining behind the curtains (or trying to?), imagine something enjoyable you'll do today or at the weekend, and think that you'll soon have that first delicious glass of juice, cup of tea or toast and jam.

There's always a light and dark side to everything, which is why it's important to be optimistic and open about life. But for that, you need to be healthy, both physically and in mind and spirit. One of my favourite quotes is from the great Oscar Wilde: 'To love oneself is the beginning of a lifelong romance.' Isn't that beautiful and so *true*? You *must* love, or at least *like* yourself and what you have achieved, otherwise if you won't, who will?

You may think, 'Oh, I haven't achieved much,' but you have. You achieved growing up and having relationships with people, with your family and friends. Count your friends. I'll bet you have a lot more than you think you have, but of course, it's relative. The Queen may have many more friends than you but maybe the woman who lives down the street has less. You achieved learning – even if you didn't pass 'A' levels you know how to read, write, talk, argue, discuss, evaluate, bargain, catch a bus, plan a holiday, cook a meal, change a light bulb. Tiny things, true, but each an achievement in its own way.

I often have truly negative articles written about me, in which my achievements are sneeringly dismissed. So what do I do when I read this rubbish? Most of the time I ignore it, but occasionally it can be so arbitrarily vicious that I sit and think about myself for a while. I compare what I have done and accomplished in my life with the writer, usually someone who hasn't ever written a book, appeared in a film or play, given birth to children or had a loving relationship, and certainly not someone who has continued to have a successful career for decades.

I'm proud of my achievements. Even though I don't have an Oscar and a string of great films to my credit, I am an optimistic,

WITH AGE COMES WISDOM | 219

happy, healthy, contented human being, who has never stopped living and working; I've supported myself and my children, and I believe that is my most major achievement and my power. And you, too, are more powerful than you think. You have the potential to achieve and enjoy more, and you must never give up. When, in 1996, I won the case against Random House everyone asked me if I would ever work again. 'Of course,' I replied, 'the opinion of a bunch of opinionated misogynists who wanted to make an example of me because they have been stupidly paying their other writers too much money won't deter me.' And it didn't. In fact, it made me more determined than ever to write, and I began writing more and more.

Certainly it was upsetting, but, like Mae West said, 'Any time you get upset, it tears down your nervous system.' I decided to believe I was strong enough not to allow myself to be frightened by those petty little publishers, and thoughts are powerful weapons. Every creative act we do begins with a thought. Your mind is super-powerful, use it.

I *knew* I was a good writer because I'd already had several bestselling books published, but I also knew it was necessary to take another tack from writing books. I took the opportunity to write an occasional diary column for *The Spectator*, an upmarket, some may call it elitist, weekly magazine, written and read by intelligent people whose opinions I respect. From my diaries I gained a great deal of approbation and also more confidence. Now I'm writing more than ever. So thanks, Random House!

So there you have them. My ways of dealing with, coping with, enjoying and loving this life of mine, which I appreciate more each passing day. When Anthony Newley sang 'The World is Full of Beautiful Things' in *Dr Doolittle*, I was married to him at the time and the words didn't mean a damn thing to me. Now, when I watch him perform it in a re-run on television and listen to those words, they have a whole new meaning for me because I believe I understand the wonder of life and with each year I love it more.

So you're getting older, so what? It's better than the only other known alternative, isn't it? Enjoy yourself now because it's later than you think!

Exhausted after writing this tome, the author relaxes in typical laid-back fashion.

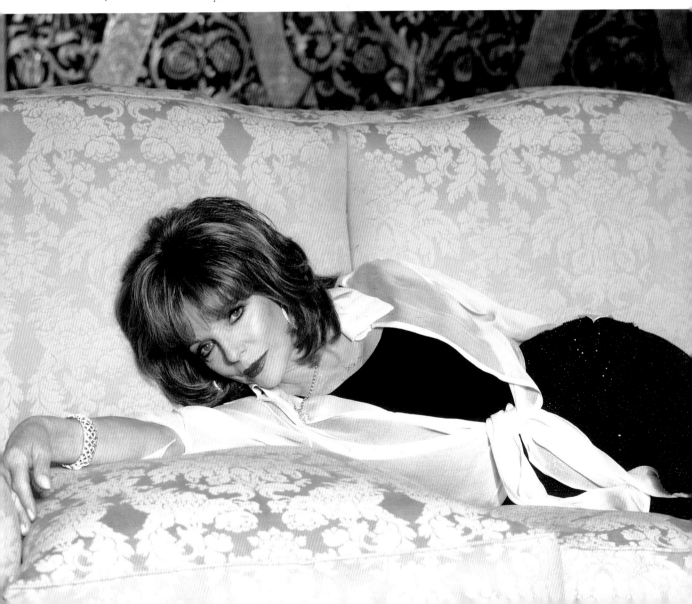

Bibliography

Airola, Dr. Paavo. *Worldwide Secrets for Staying Young*.
HEALTH PLUS PUBLISHERS, 1982

Ducket, Suzanne and Stapely, Tabitha. *The Spa Directory*.
CARLTON, 2002.

Edgson, Vicki and Marber, Ian. *The Food Doctor: Healing Foods for Mind and Body*.
COLLINS & BROWN, 1999.

Edgson, Vicki and Marber, Ian. *In Bed with The Food Doctor: How to Eat Your Way to Better Sex and Sleep*.
COLLINS & BROWN, 2001.

Gill, AA. *The Ivy: The Restaurant and its Recipes*.
HODDER & STOUGHTON, 1997.

Gill, AA. *Le Caprice*.
HODDER & STOUGHTON, 1999.

Klatz, Dr. Ronald and Goldman, Dr. Robert. *Stopping the Clock: Dramatic Breakthroughs in Anti-Aging and Age Reversal Techniques*.
BANTAM BOOKS, 1997.

Lowe, Professor Nicolas and Sellar, Polly. *Skin Secrets: The Medical Facts Versus the Beauty Fiction*.
COLLINS & BROWN, 1999.

Rosenfeld, Isadore, MD. *Live Now, Age Later: Proven Ways to Slow Down the Clock*.
WARNER BOOKS, 1999.

Selby, Anna. *The Juice and Zest Book*.
COLLINS & BROWN, 2000.

Index

Acknowledgements

I would like to thank my wonderfully supportive publisher and hands-on editor, Jeremy Robson, for his devoted support for this book; also Jane Donovan for her dedicated editing and Ian Hughes, who executed the superb layouts to great effect.

Brian Aris, photographer *par excellence*, helped me tremendously, not only with his calmness and expertise in the taking of many photographs but in his choice of his archival material and canny knowledge of what pictures would improve each layout.

Grateful thanks to Paul Keylock for his endless patience in being able to source ancient and modern photographs of me. To Wolfgang Puck, Sirio Maccioni, Yvonne Fravola, The Ivy and Le Caprice for sharing with me some of their succulent recipes. To Sally Bulloch at The Athenaeum, Piccadilly, and Ellen Spann at Claridge's, Mayfair, where a number of the photos for this book were taken, and to OK! Magazine for allowing me to reproduce a selection of my wedding photos. And thanks to my agent, Jonathan Lloyd, who really cares (unlike many of them!).

And last, but by no means least, I want to thank my husband, Percy Gibson. With his knowledge of the power of the Internet and his proficiency with his word processor and computer, he has helped and encouraged me immeasurably.

Robson Books would like to thank Matthew Archer, Jan Archibald, Christine Bernstein, Tonia Czerniawskyi, David Downton, Scott Del Amo/Cobra, Richard Emerson, Terry Forshaw, Highclere Castle, David Hooper, Gill and Zoë Hughes, Warren Keogan, Alison Leach, Norma Macmillan, Eddie Sanderson, Pam Sharp and Richard Young.

Frederick Fox of Mayfair, hatmaker to HM The Queen, kindly supplied the pillbox hat featured on page 147.

Special thanks to Grayshott Hall Health Fitness Retreat for their hospitality and for providing the location for photography on pages 23, 49, 89, 138 and 140.

For further information, contact:
Grayshott Hall Health Fitness Retreat, Headley Road
Grayshott near Hindhead, Surrey TU26 6JJ
Telephone: 01428 602000

Picture credits
All photos including cover by Brian Aris © Robson Books with the exception of the following: Half title: Portrait of Joan Collins by David Downton; title page, pp13, 119 and 146 (top and bottom) from These Old Broads, photographer Wayne Massarelli, © Columbia Tristar Television; pp5 (top), 63, 96, 113, 122, 207, back cover (bottom photo) and back flap of cover (second from top) © Brian Aris Archive; pp5 (bottom), 16, 45, 90, 92, 98, 108, 109, 110 (left), 111, 128, 130, 137, 146 (bottom), 160, 166, 173, 187, 193 (bottom left), 197, 202, 204, 211, 224 and front flap of cover (bottom photo) from the private collection of Joan Collins; pp15, 16, 28, 81 and 203 from the personal collection of Paul Keylock; pp17 and 213 © Scott Del Amo/Cobra; pp29, 115 and 129 © Richard Young/Rex Features; page 39 © Paramount Pictures Television; page 91 all photos © UPPA; page 99 © Eddie Sanderson. On location Empire of the Ants and pp121 and 151; page 100 © Chris Barham; pp110 (right), 112, 169 (left) Michael Barnett/The Kobal Collection; page 116 © Private collection of Rene Horsch; page 125 © Universal Pictures Flintstones Viva Rock Vegas; pp167, 175, 191, 193 (above and bottom right), 197 and front flap of cover (second from top) photos by Brian Aris/© OK! Magazine; page 169 (right) Gerard Decaux/Rex; page 172 The Kobal Collection; page 183 © Dennis Stone; back flap of cover (third from top) © Universal Pictures.